DATE			

MEDICAL
INTELLIGENCE
UNIT

THE THYMUS—

REGULATOR OF CELLULAR IMMUNITY

John A. Goss, M.D.
M. Wayne Flye, M.D., Ph.D.

Washington University
St. Louis

R.G. LANDES COMPANY
AUSTIN

MEDICAL INTELLIGENCE UNIT

THE THYMUS—REGULATOR OF CELLULAR IMMUNITY

R.G. LANDES COMPANY
Austin

CRC Press is the exclusive worldwide distributor of publications of the Medical Intelligence Unit.
CRC Press, 2000 Corporate Blvd., NW, Boca Raton, FL 33431. Phone: 407/994-0555.

Submitted: August 1993
Published: October 1993

Production Manager: Terry Nelson
Copy Editor: Constance Kerkaporta

Please address all inquiries to the Publisher:
R.G. Landes Company, 909 Pine Street, Georgetown, TX 78626
or
P.O. Box 4858, Austin, TX 78765
Phone: 512/ 863 7762; FAX: 512/ 863 0081

ISBN 1-879702-81-9
CATALOG # LN0281

Libary of Congress Cataloging-in-Publication Data
Goss, John A.
The thymus : regulator of cellular immunity / John A. Goss, M. Wayne Flye.
p. cm.—(Medical intelligence unit)
Includes bibliographical references and index.
ISBN 1-879702-81-9 : $89.95
1. Thymus—Physiology. 2. Cellular immunity. I. Flye, M. Wayne. II. Title. III. Series.
[DNLM: 1. Thymus Gland—anatomy & histology. 2. Thymus Gland-physiolgy. 3. T-Lymphocytes—physiology . T-Lymphocytes—immunology. WK 400 G677t 1993]
QR185.8.T48G67 1993
612.4'3—dc20
DNLM/DLC
for Library of Congress
93-35864
CIP

CONTENTS

PREFACE

In recent years, organ transplantation has gone from the realm of experimental medicine to the standard of care for isolated end-stage organ failure. However, Peter Medawar early recognized that rejection directed against the transplantation antigens was the principle barrier to the ultimate success of the therapeutic approach. Pharmacologic advances in nonspecific immunosuppression and technical advances in solid organ transplantation have improved the survival results of kidney, liver, heart, lung and pancreas allografts over the last decade. Transplantation biologists have long recognized that the complications of long-term immunosuppression could be avoided if it were possible to achieve a state of donor-specific unresponsiveness without immunosuppression, as was achieved by Billingham et al in murine neonatal tolerance. The achievement of this state of tolerance appears to depend upon the presentation of antigen before the development of a competent T cell repertoire, thus allowing developing T cells to recognize the foreign antigen as self and thereby to specifically delete reactive T cell clones.

While not a comprehensive discussion of all methods of tolerance induction for allograft transplantation, this monograph intends to provide the reader with an overview of the anatomy and physiology of the mammalian thymus and the current understanding of T lymphocyte maturation, and its restriction by the major histocompatibility complex. Because of the interest of our laboratory in attempting to define the role of the thymus in the development of allograft tolerance, detailed experiments centering on the thymus during the induction of donor-specific allograft tolerance are described. The complexity of the biology of allograft rejection, with many as yet unknown variables, excites the interest of the transplantation community in the role of the thymus in the development of tolerance to allo- and possibly xenografts, and especially the mechanisms of intrathymic antigen-induced tolerance and its possible application to clinical transplantation.

Acknowledgments

The authors would like to express their gratitude to Mrs. Theresa Belgeri for her tireless secretarial assistance in the preparation of this monograph.

CHAPTER 1

INTRODUCTION

Although the thymic structure was recognized by the Greeks, the function of this gland remained enigmatic until comparatively recently when the science of immunology began to elucidate the origin and function of peripheral lymphocytes in disease. The thymus is a bilobed lymphoid organ which develops from a paired epithelial anlage in the neck and descends to the superior mediastinum. At the completion of this descent, the thymus is located in the anterior aspect of the thoracic cavity and lower part of the neck, anterior to the great vessels originating from the aortic arch. During embryological development the thymus is the first lymphoid organ to appear. The major activity of the thymus occurs during childhood after which it gradually involutes such that, in adult humans, the thymus is often impossible to differentiate from the surrounding connective tissue. The thymus is embryologically derived from epithelial outgrowths of the primitive pharynx, and monoclonal antibody studies have determined that precursors of $\alpha\beta$ and $\gamma\delta$ T-cell-receptor (TCR) bearing T cells which are derived from hematopoietic tissue developing elsewhere in the embryo colonize the primitive thymus on approximately day 11 and 14.5 of fetal life respectively. The principal functions of the thymus include the reception of hematopoietic precursors, the subsequent maturation and/or selection of antigen specific T cells, and the selective release of such cells to constitute the peripheral lymphoid repertoire.

The maturation of T (thymus-derived) cells in the thymus involves the successive induction of a remarkable array of lineage-restricted genes, some of which are expressed only during the intrathymic phase of differentiation, and others whose expression is maintained throughout the T cell's life span. During thymocyte and T-cell maturation, genes encoding the TCR α and β or δ and γ chains rearrange and are then expressed at the cell surface as receptor heterodimers. These events precede or accompany the expression of the CD4 and CD8 molecules, which enable the selection of T cells that recognize the products of thymic-specific MHC gene products necessary for immune cell interaction. During thymic residence T cells acquire the ability to provide help to antibody-producing B cells, to kill allospecific targets and to suppress immune responses. At a later stage of intrathymic maturation, the developing thymocyte acquires functional levels of cell surface homing receptors, such as MEL-14 and LPAM-1, which appear to be responsible for the specific migration of mature lymphocytes from the bloodstream into organized peripheral lymphoid tissues.

This monograph is designed to provide an overview of intrathymic anatomy and physiology in the regulation of cellular immunity. We have summarized our current understanding of these concepts and what part they may play in the development of tolerance to "self" and alloantigens. However, our knowledge of intra- and extrathymic T-cell development and MHC restriction is rapidly growing. While it is apparent that the thymus occupies a central position in regulating T-cell development, its role at the cellular and molecular level has yet to be precisely defined. The first portion of this monograph will outline the basic anatomy and physiology of the mammalian thymus and will include reviews of its embryology, gross anatomy, microanatomy, microenvironment, and the cytokines and hormones produced by the thymus. The second portion will attempt to apply this knowledge to the explanation of clinical entities such as thymic hypoplasia, T-cell ontogeny, the role of the CD4 and CD8 accessory cell surface molecules during the differentiation of thymocytes, as well as the development of MHC restriction, "self" tolerance and the development of tolerance to alloantigens. Because of the interest of our laboratory in attempting to understand the role played by the thymus in the development of allograft tolerance, our detailed studies centering on the thymus during the induction of donor-specific allograft tolerance are presented.

HISTORICAL PERSPECTIVE

The name "thymus" is derived from one of two differently accented Greek words meaning an herb, or the heart or soul. Many medieval students regarded the thymus as at the heart of good health. It is reputed that Galen, who lived about 130-200 A.D., first described the morphology of the thymus gland and it attracted sporadic interest ever since, particularly in the 1900s when hyperplasia was noted to occur in conjunction with myasthenia gravis. In 1901, Laquer and Weigert[1] in Frankfurt provided the first description of a tumor in a patient suffering from myasthenia gravis; no connection between the thymus gland and myasthenia had previously been suggested. For many years, association with a thymic tumor remained nothing more than an observation. Since removal of the tumor was not surgically feasible, the whole subject of diagnosis and treatment of myasthenia gravis was hardly mentioned because there was no treatment. In 1911, Sauerbruch[2] performed the first thymectomy in a patient suffering from both myasthenia and hyperthyroidism, with a view to improving the thyroid condition. Since this failed, a thyroidectomy was subsequently performed with more effect, but the myasthenia was incidentally improved, suggesting a possible connection between myasthenia and thymic disease. Nevertheless, it was many years before Blalock (Fig. 1) in 1936,[3] by removal of a thymic tumor, successfully treated myasthenia in a young female patient who had previously failed radiotherapy to the thymus. He reported the result of his operation in 1939,[3] and two years later took a second critical step when he removed the entire thymus from six myasthenic patients. All of the patients recovered and the results of these operations were reported in preliminary fashion in 1941,[4] and the results of his first 20 patients were reported in detail in 1944.[5] These reports represent the beginning of modern surgical therapy for myasthenia gravis and confirmed the association of thymic tumors and myasthenia gravis, thereby laying the foundations for the modern ideas on the recognition and treatment of thymic tumors.[7,8]

In the early 1930s, it was thought that babies and young children often suffered (and were thought to die) from an enlarged thymus (status thymicolymphaticus).[9,10] By the late 1930s this condition had been thoroughly examined and was no longer accepted as a disease entity. However, these studies resulted in many records of thymic weight and size in fetuses, children, and adults[11,12,13,14] which have until recently formed the basis of our understanding of thymic size, weight, and immunologic activity in adult life. Of necessity, many of the data were taken from maximally stressed

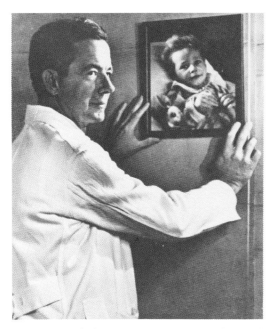

Fig. 1. Dr. Alfred Blalock, 1899-1964, Professor of Surgery at Vanderbilt University and Johns Hopkins Hospital, pioneered thymectomy for myasthenia gravis. [From Ravitch MM. 1946. In: A Century of Surgery 1880-1980. Philadelphia, Toronto: JB Lippincott, 1981:891.]

patients dying from terminal illness after long-term hospitalization. Although the authors were aware that the patients studied were not healthy, they were not aware of the thymic involution that would occur, resulting in a vast underestimation of the size and activity of the adult thymus.[15]

Thus, although the thymus was studied during and after disease, no specific role was attributed to it in health. Indeed, it was thought to be an unnecessary organ, and with the development of cardiac surgery, part or all of the thymus was indiscriminately removed in patients of all ages to provide surgical exposure.[16] Not only was it demonstrated that adults could survive thymectomy, but the gland was often found at postmortem examination to have atrophied in adults. In neonatal mice, however, its presence appeared vital, as animals thymectomized around the time of birth died of wasting or runts' disease, secondary to degranulation of the anterior pituitary growth hormone and loss of prolactin production.[17] More recently, it was realized that the gland also has an important role early in the development of sexual organs. Infants with little or no thymus at birth, e.g., DiGeorge and *cri du chat* syndromes, and ataxia telangiectasia, all fail to develop normal gonads, secondary to the lack of the thymic hormone, thymosin, which stimulates the secretion of luteinizing hormone releasing hormone from the hypothalamus.[18]

After Glick, Chang, and Japp in 1956[19] identified the bursa of Fabricius in birds as the source of antibody-producing B (bursa-derived) cells, circulating lymphocytes were divided into T and B cells.[20] While no bursa equivalent was identified in mammals, it was appreciated that the thymus allowed the generation of T cells. This elicited intense research interest in thymocytes and the thymic microenvironment. A major focus was that T cells appeared to be devoid of receptors for antigen, equivalent to B-cell immunoglobulins.

Today, the structure of T-cell receptors (TCR) is known in great detail[21,22] and their study is of critical importance to immunological research. It is now generally accepted that selection processes during T-cell differentiation are responsible for the survival of thymocytes which express only "useful" TCRs, i.e., TCRs that recognize foreign antigens in association with self-major histocompatibility complex (MHC) molecules. The

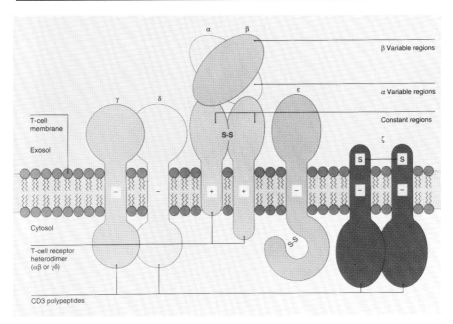

Fig. 2. Diagramatic representation of the T-cell antigen receptor heterodimer (αβ or γδ) with the four distinct CD3 polypeptides. [From Davis MM. 1988. Molecular genetics of T-cell antigen receptors. Hosp Pract 1988;15:157-170.]

postthymic T-cell repertoire appears to arise from a subset of thymocytes which have TCR-binding affinity for the particular MHC molecules expressed in the thymus.[23,24] The TCR (Fig. 2) is a heterodimer composed of three polypeptide chains [the cell differentiation marker 3 (CD3)] closely associated with a disulfide-linked dimer (either an α and a β chain or a γ and a δ chain). This TCR has an exposed groove into which may fit the antigenic determinants of the major histocompatibility complex.[25,26] The TCR in conjunction with CD4 surface molecules (CD4+ T helper cells) recognizes MHC class II, and in conjunction with CD8 surface molecules (CD8+ T suppressor/cytotoxic cells) recognizes MHC class I molecules. Different T cells can, therefore, be regarded as restricted to their recognition of foreign antigen in combination with self MHC antigens. The results of their interaction with antigen in the periphery is T-cell activation, with resulting expression of factors, such as interleukin-2 (IL-2) and its receptor, which in turn results in T-cell proliferation and clonal expansion.

The in vivo control of the developmental sequences of differentiating thymocytes is considered to be under the influence of the thymic microenvironment. Many events can influence this microenvironment. Some can be physiologic changes throughout life, such as aging and pregnancy; others are viral infections, thymomas, or stress. Recently emphasis has been directed to the exquisite sensitivity of the thymus for natural immunotoxins[27] and, therefore, environmental or man-made insults must also be considered. However, this monograph is largely restricted to reviewing our current concept of the influence of the thymus on T-cell differentiation, MHC restriction, the development of self tolerance, and how the role of the thymus can be manipulated during the induction of donor specific allograft tolerance.

REFERENCES

1. Laquer L, Weigert C. Beitrage zur lehre von der erb'schen krankheit. Neurol Centralbl 1901; 20: 594-98.
2. Schumacher ED, Roth J. Thymektomie bei einem Fall von Morbus Basedowi mit Myasthenie. Mitteilungen Grenzgebeiten der Medizin und Chirurgie 1912; 25: 746-65.
3. Blalock A, Mason MF, Morgan HJ, Riven SS. Myasthenia gravis and tumors of the thymic region: Report of a case in which the tumor was removed. Ann Surg 1939; 110: 544.
4. Blalock A, Harvey AM, Ford FR, Lilienthal JL Jr. The treatment of myasthenia gravis by removal of the thymus gland: Preliminary report. J Amer Med Assoc 1941; 117: 1529.
5. Blalock A. Thymectomy in the treatment of myasthenia gravis: Report of 20 cases. J Thorac Surg 1944; 13: 316.
6. Keynes G. The results of thymectomy in myasthenia gravis. Br Med J (Clinical research) ii. 1949; 611-16.
7. Keynes G. Investigations into thymic disease and tumor formation. Br J Surg 1955; 42: 449-62.
8. Keynes G. In: The Gates of Memory. Oxford: Clarendon, 1982: 273-84.
9. Boyd E. Growth of the thymus: Its relation to status lymphaticus and thymic symptoms. Am J Dis Child 1927; 33: 867.
10. Cooperstock M. Present concepts of enlarged thymus and status lymphaticus: Review of a decade of experience. J Michigan Med Soc 1930; 29: 21.
11. Bratton AB. The normal weight of the human thymus. J Path Bacter 1925; 28: 609-20.
12. Greenwood M, Woods HM. "Status thymico-lymphaticus" considered in the light of recent work on the thymus. J Hygiene (London) 1927; 26: 305-26.
13. Scammon RE. The prenatal growth of the human thymus. Proc Soci Exp Biol Med 1927; 24: 906-09.
14. Young M, Turnbull HM. An analysis of the data collected by the status lymphaticus investigation committee. J Pathol Bacter 1931; 34: 213-58.
15. Kendall MD, Johnson HRM, Singh J. The weight of the human thymus gland at necropsy. J Anat 1980; 131: 485-99.
16. Zollinger RM, Jr., Lindem MC, Filler RM, Corson JM, Wilson RE. Effect of thymectomy on skin-homograft survival in children. N Engl J Med 1964; 270: 707.
17. Bianchi E, Pierpaoli W, Sorkin E. Cytological changes in the mouse anterior pituitary after neonatal thymectomy: A light and electron microscopical study. J Endocrin 1971; 51: 1.
18. Rebar RW, Miyake A, Low TLK, Goldstein AL. Thymosin stimulates secretion of luteinizing hormone-releasing factor. Science 1981; 214: 669.
19. Glick B, Chang TS, & Japp RG. The bursa of Fabricius and antibody production. Poultry Science 1956; 35: 224-25.
20. Szenberg A, Warner NL. Immunological functions of the thymus and bursa of fabricius. Disassociation of immunological responsiveness in fowls with a hormonally arrested development of lymphoid tissues. Nature 1962; 194: 146-47.
21. Travers P. One hand clapping. Nature 1990; 348: 393-94.

22. Finkel TH, Kubo RT, Cambier JC. T-cell development and transmembrane signaling: changing biological responses through an unchanging receptor. Immunology Today 1991; 12: 79-85.

23. Teh HS, Kisielow P, Scott B, et al. Thymic major histocompatibility antigens and the αβ T-cell receptor determine the CD4/CD8 phenotype of T cells. Nature 1988; 335: 229.

24. Sha WC, Nelson CA, Newberry RD, et al. Positive and negative selection of an antigen receptor on T cells in transgenic mice. Nature 1988; 336: 73.

25. Salter RD, Benjamin RJ, Wesley PK, et al. A binding site for the T-cell coreceptor CD8 on the α 3 domain of HLA-A2. Nature 1990; 345: 41-46.

26. Wang J, Yan Y, Garrett TPJ, et al. Atomic structure of a fragment of human CD4 containing two immunoglobulin-like domains. Nature 1990; 348: 411-18.

27. Kendall MD, Ritter MA. The thymus in immunotoxicology. Thymus Update 4. London: Harwood Academic, 1991: 267-94.

CHAPTER 3

DEVELOPMENTAL ANATOMY

The first definitive studies of the anatomic development of the pharyngeal pouch derivatives are those of Weller[1] and Norris.[2] In mammals the thymus gland, along with the inferior parathyroid glands, develop from the ventral diverticula of the third branchial pouch, with an inconstant contribution from the fourth branchial pouch during the sixth intrauterine week (Fig. 1 and 2).[3] At the end of the sixth gestational week the third branchial pouch develops a pronounced ventral sacculation and separates from the pharynx (Fig. 3).[4] At this time the third branchial pouch is in contact with the fourth branchial cleft, which has itself lost its connection with the surface ectoderm. From the dorsal portion of the third branchial pouch, the inferior parathyroid glands differentiate. Initially the thymic primordium are hollow and retain a lumen, the thymopharyngeal duct which is a derivative of the third branchial pouch, but subsequently rapidly undergoes differentiation to become solid epithelial bars (Fig. 4). The epithelium of this duct is endodermal, and there is possibly an ectodermal contribution from the fourth branchial cleft. The parathyroids unlike the thymic primordium are solid from their first appearance when they are differentiating into their distinctive clear cells.

During the seventh and eighth gestational weeks the thymuses elongate and enlarge caudally and anterolaterally. The end of the eighth gestational week marks the fusion of the advancing distal ends of the thymic primordia at the level of the superior margin of the aortic arch and the loss of its connection with the branchial clefts (Fig. 5).[1] This midline fusion affects only the connective tissue since the parenchyma does not fuse and, therefore, never truly loses its paired nature.[3] At the completion of this fusion, the most caudal end of the thymus enlarges and attaches to the pericardium which dictates the thymus' permanent position in the anterior-superior mediastinum. During this dissent into the thorax there is an accompanying change in the relative growth rates of the cranial and caudal portions of the thymuses, so that the caudal portion differentiates and proliferates at a much more rapid rate and eventually becomes much thicker than the cranial portion.[5] The cephalic connections with the pharynx disappear during the eighth gestational week, leaving the definitive thymus in the mediastinum. Cervical thymic cysts or small islands of thymic tissue may be found in ectopic locations such as the tympanic cavity, neck, mediastinum or lung from persistent remnants of the tubular upper end of the primitive organ (Fig. 6).[6] Aberrant (ectopic) nodules of thymic tissue are found in approximately 20% of humans.[7] These islands of ectopic thymic tissue can be the site of origin of pathologic conditions including hyperplastic lesions, cysts and tumors.

The thymus is the first of the lymphoid organs to develop and it has essentially matured between the 15th and 20th gestational weeks.[8,9] The development of normal peripheral lymph nodes depend on subsequent seeding by small lymphocytes from the thymus. This is emphasized in patients with DiGeorge syndrome (thymic aplasia), where lymph nodes with germinal centers are found, but contain few lymphocytes. In severe combined immunodeficiency disease, lymph nodes contain reticulum cells only.

Until the seventh gestational week, the thymus is an epithelial organ and only undifferentiated epithelial cells are present. This cell mass becomes invaded by mesenchyme containing the lymphocytic stem cells. There is

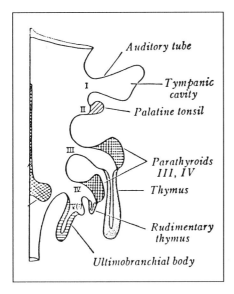

Fig. 1. The human pharynx and its derivatives in ventral outline at six weeks gestational age. [From L.B. Arey. The Pharynx. In: Developmental Anatomy, 7th ed., Philadelphia: Saunders, 1965: 196]

Fig. 2. Pharynx with right third and fourth branchial pouches at 6th gestational week. [From L.B. Arey. The Pharynx. In: Developmental Anatomy, 7th ed., Philadelphia: Saunders, 1965: 198]

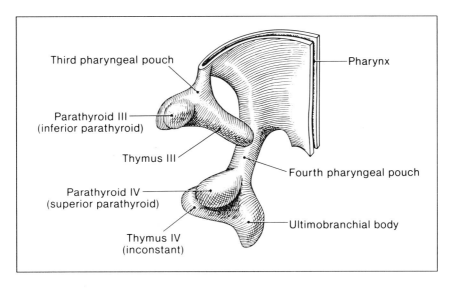

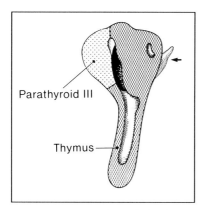

Fig. 3. Long section through the derivatives of the third branchial pouch at the 6th gestational week. The ventral (thymic) portion retains a lumen. The arrow indicates the point of detachment from the pharynx. [From L.B. Arey. The Pharynx. In: Developmental Anatomy, 7th ed., Philadelphia: Saunders, 1965: 198]

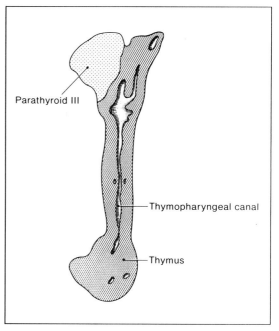

Fig. 4. (Above, right) Elongation of the thymic portion of the third branchial pouch derivative at the 8th gestational week. The thymopharyngeal canal is disappearing. [From L.B. Arey. The Pharynx. In: Developmental Anatomy, 7th ed., Philadelphia: Saunders, 1965: 198]

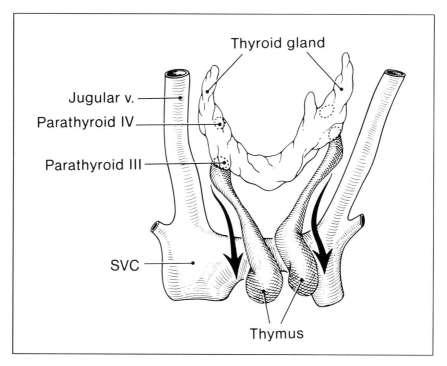

Fig. 5. The descent of the thymus at the end of the second month. The cranial ends of the thymus will disappear; the descending caudal ends will form the definitive thymus. SVC—superior vena cava. [From L.B. Arey. The Pharynx. In: Developmental Anatomy, 7th ed., Philadelphia: Saunders, 1965: 199]

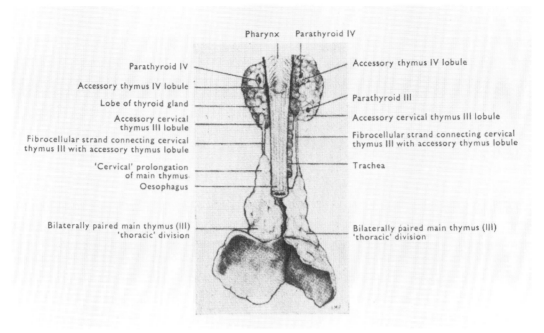

Pharynx   Parathyroid IV

Parathyroid IV

Accessory thymus IV lobule

Lobe of thyroid gland

Accessory cervical thymus III lobule

Fibrocellular strand connecting cervical thymus III with accessory thymus lobule

'Cervical' prolongation of main thymus
Oesophagus

Bilaterally paired main thymus (III) 'thoracic' division

Accessory thymus IV lobule

Parathyroid III

Accessory cervical thymus III lobule

Fibrocellular strand connecting cervical thymus III with accessory thymus lobule

Trachea

Bilaterally paired main thymus (III) 'thoracic' division

Fig. 6. Illustration of accessory thymic lobules described by Groschuff (1900). [From RG Harrison. The Ductless Glands. In: GJ Romanes, ed. Cunningham's Textbook of Anatomy, Oxford, New York, Toronto: Oxford University Press, 1981: 602.]

evidence from chick embryos that the neural crest may act as an organizer of an interaction between the epithelial primordium and the invading mesenchyme.[10] Whereas the neural crest cells themselves contribute only to the development of the connective tissues of the thymic septa and blood vessels, neural crest mesoectoderm contributes to thymus formation via interaction with ectoderm from pharyngeal pouches III and IV, and to tissues that subsequently differentiate to support thymopoiesis. The mesenchyme of the aortic arches is also derived from neural crest, and the truncal septum also contains neural crest cells. The significance of this common origin is that developmental abnormalities of neural crest derivatives affect the formation of the heart, the thymus and the peripheral ganglia. Couly et al[11] have proposed this explanation for the DiGeorge and Pierre Robin syndromes, where the absence or hypoplasia of the thymus is associated with cardiac malformations.

During the 8th to 10th gestational week, the thymus begins to attract hematopoietic stem cells before vascularization of the organ has occurred. In avian and murine chimeras, waves of stem cells enter at restricted times of embryonic and possibly postnatal life.[12,13] These prethymic stem cells initially originate extraembryonically from the yolk sac, later from the fetal liver, and in neonates and adults from the bone marrow. In mice, cells capable of colonizing pharyngeal pouch tissues in culture are negative for the THY-1 thymocyte marker and are probably spleen colony forming units (CFU-S). However, the degree of multipotentiality of prethymic stem cells has not been resolved, especially since different waves of immigrants (from

Table 1. Chronology of the developing mammalian thymus

Developmental Event	Gestational Week
Pouch III Formed	5th
Elongation of Epithelial Primordia	7th-8th
Invasion of Mesenchyme	7th
Disappearance of Cephalic Portion,	8th
Descent of Thymus	8th
Stem Cells in Thymus	8th-10th
Lobes Visible	9th
Hassel's Corpuscles Present	11th
Cortex and Medulla Defined	12th-17th
Thymus Mature	15th-20th
Greatest Size of Thymus	Puberty

different sources at various times throughout life) may have preexisting restrictions on their multipotency.

Thymus lobes begin to appear in the 9th to 12th gestational weeks in man. Septa from the mesenchyme around the primordium begins to indent the layer of epithelial cells and create an "opening" in the capsule which advances to the corticomedullary junction as the medulla begins to form around 14 weeks of gestation. This structural change allows other cells such as monocytes to enter and become the interdigitating cells of the medulla and for nerves and blood vessels to travel through the septa into the medulla. Although blood vessels do pass into the parenchyma of the gland, they are always surrounded by subcapsular epithelium in the cortex and partly so in the medulla.[14,15]

Medullary epithelial cells are morphologically distinct from other thymic epithelial cells and the medulla, which is fully formed by 17 weeks of gestation, contains a different population of thymocytes and accessory cells than in the cortex. Although it is believed that pharyngeal epithelial cells eventually give rise to at least some of the defined epithelial cell classes within the thymus,[16] definitive marker experiments allowing identification of the endodermal, ectodermal and mesenchymal cells have not yet been performed in mammals.

The means by which precursor T lymphocytes leave blood vessels and reach the thymic microenvironment remains obscure. There is evidence that during specific intervals, the developing thymic microenvironment sends out signals that attract thymus homing hematopoietic cells. During embryonic life, waves of cells then enter the thymus and establish self-renewing and differentiating lines of thymic lymphocytes.[17] It has also been shown that, after the neonatal period, lymphocytes in S phase home to the thymus with a higher frequency than do resting or blasted lymphocytes.[18,19,20]

The origin and significance of Hassel's corpuscles, small bodies of flattened epithelial cells arranged around a granular nucleated cell found in the thymic medulla, are not clear. They are not present in the early stage of thymic development. There is evidence that they are remnants of endodermal origin in epithelial cords around which the mesenchymal portion develops.[21] Similarities and possibly a common origin between Hassel's corpuscles and epidermal keratinocytes have been pointed out[22] by electron microscopic and histochemical methods.

The thymus grows rapidly during embryonic life, and in the neonatal period reaches its largest relative size.[23] However, the human thymus reaches its greatest absolute size at puberty (approximately 35 grams)[24] and then undergoes slow involution, although nonatrophic portions may continue to function normally for many years. With aging, total lymphoid mass is lost, much of the thymus is replaced by fat, and both cortical lymphocytes and T lymphocytes in the peripheral blood are reduced. Table 1 recapitulates the development of the thymus.

REFERENCES

1. Weller GJ. Development of the thyroid, parathyroid, and thymus glands in man. Contrib Embryol 1933; 24: 93-142.
2. Norris EH. The parathyroid glands and the lateral thyroid in man: their morphogenesis, histogenesis, topographic anatomy and prenatal growth. Contrib Embryol 1937; 26: 247-94.
3. Siegler R. The thymus and the unicorn—two great myths of gross anatomy. Anat Rec 1969; 163: 264-97.
4. Norris EH. The morphogenesis and histogenesis of the thymus gland in man. Contrib Embryol 1938; 27: 191-208.
5. Hamilton WJ, Mossman HW. Embryology of the Alimentary and Respiratory Systems, Pleural and Peritoneal cavities. In: Hamilton WJ, Mossman HW, eds Human Embryology: Prenatal Development of Form and Function. 4th ed. Baltimore: Williams and Williams, 1972: 315-18.
6. Rosai J, Levine GD. Tumors of the thymus. In: Fascille B, ed. Atlas of Tumor Pathology, Second Series. Washington: Armed Forces Institute of Pathology, 1976.
7. Gilmour JR. Some developmental abnormalities of the thymus and parathyroids. J Pathol Bacteriol 1941; 52: 13-19.
8. Haynes B. Phenotypic characterization and ontogeny of components of the human thymic microenvironment. Clin Res 1984; 32: 500-07.
9. Papiernik M. Ontogeny of the human lymphoid system: study of the cytological maturation and the incorporation of tritiated thymidine and uridine in the fetal thymus and lymph node and in the infantile thymus. J Cell Physiol 1972; 80: 235-42.
10. Bockman D, Kirby ML. Dependence of thymus development on derivatives of the neural crest. Science 1984; 223: 498-500.
11. Couly G, LaGrue A, Griscelli C. Le Syndrome de DiGeorge, neurocristopathie rhombencephalique exemplaire. Rev Stromatol Chir Maxillofac 1983; 84: 103-07.
12. Moore M, Metcalf D. Ontogeny of the hematopoietic system: Yolk sac origin of in vivo and in vitro colony forming cells in the developing mouse embryo. Br J Hematol 1970; 18: 279-96.
13. Fontaine-Perus JC, Culman FM, Kaplan C, et al. Seeding of the 10-day mouse embryo thymic rudiment by lymphocyte precursors in vitro. J Immunol 1981; 126: 2310-16.
14. Raitsina S, Kalinina II. Differentiation of thymic lymphoid cells during human embryogenesis. Dev Comp Immunol 1984; 8: 225-30.

15. Kendall MD. The morphology of the perivascular spaces. Thymus 1989; 13: 157-64.
16. Von Gaudecker B, Muller-Hermelink HK. Ontogeny and organization of the stationary nonlymphoid cells in the human thymus. Cell Tissue Res 1980; 207: 287-306.
17. Jotereau F, Heuze F, Salomon-Vie V, Gascan H. Cell kinetics in the fetal mouse thymus: Precursor cell input, proliferation, and emigration. J Immunol 1987; 138: 1026-30.
18. Michie SA, Kirkpatrick EA, Rouse RV. Rare peripheral T cells migrate to and persist in normal mouse thymus. J Exp Med 1988; 168: 1929-34.
19. Agus D, Surh CD, Sprent J. Reentry of T cells to the adult thymus is restricted to activated T cells. J Exp Med 1991; 173: 1039-46.
20. Surh CD, Sprent J, Webb SR. Exclusion of circulating T cells from the thymus does not apply in the neonatal period. J Exp Med 1993; 177: 379-85.
21. Shier K. The morphology of the epithelial thymus: observations on lymphocyte-depleted and fetal thymus. Lab Invest 1963; 12: 316-26.
22. Von Gaudecker B, Schmale EM. Similarities between Hassel's corpuscles of the human thymus and the epidermis: an investigation by electron microscopy and histochemistry. Cell Tissue Res 1974; 151: 347-68.
23. Hofmann WJ, Moller P, Otto HF. Hyperplasia. In: Groel JC, ed. Surgery of the Thymus. New York: Springer, 1990: 59-70.
24. Gray H. The Lymphatic System. In: Goss, ed. Anatomy of the Human Body. 29th ed. Philadelphia: Lea and Febiger, 1973: 772-73.

CHAPTER 4

GROSS ANATOMY

The human thymus is situated in the midline and is located predominately in the anterior (anterior-superior) mediastinum posterior to the sternothyroid and sternohyoid muscles and immediately anterior to the aortic arch and its branches, the left brachiocephalic vein, the trachea, and the pericardium. The thymus is a flattened pyramidal shaped organ composed of two closely opposed lobes (right and left), which are subdivided into a number of lobules and are held in close contact by fibrous connective tissue sheath that also encloses the entire organ in a distinct capsule (Fig. 1). However, the septa subdividing the lobes into lobules extend from the capsule and only reach the corticomedullary junction; therefore, the medulla is confluent throughout (Fig. 2).[1] The two lobes are joined in the midline by loose connective tissue at their bases, and this connection is situated just ventral to the superior extension of the pericardium. Inferiorly the thymus usually extends to the fourth costal cartilage. The superior border often reaches the caudal border of the thyroid gland but occasionally extends over the thyroid. The thymus is frequently connected to the caudal border of the thyroid gland by thin strands of connective tissue, the thyrothymic ligament, which contains several small blood vessels but little nervous tissue.[1] Occasionally the cranial limit of the thymus extends over the thyroid[2] or ectopic thymic tissue may be found in relation to the parathyroids, thyroid cartilage, tympanic cavity, and numerous mediastinal locations.[3,4] Ectopic thymus tissue is found in approximately 20-25% of humans.[5,6] These islands of ectopic thymic tissue can be the origin of pathologic conditions including hyperplastic lesions, cysts, tumors, and tumor-like lesions. Laterally the thymus lies alongside the pleura of the lung in close approximation to mediastinal fat. Anteriorly the thymus is related to the sternum, the cranial four costal cartilages, and the sternohyoid and sternothyroid muscles.[7] The cervical portion of the thymus lies ventral and lateral to the trachea, and dorsal to the origins of the sternohyoid and sternothyroid muscles. The two thymic lobes generally differ in size and shape, the right frequently being larger and overlapping the left.[8] The thymus in the human infant is pinkish-gray in color, soft and lobulated, weighs on average 13 gm, and measures approximately 5 cm in length, 4 cm in width, and 6 cm in thickness.

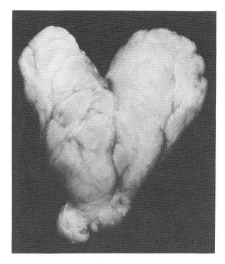 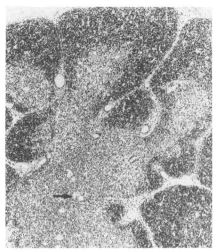

Fig. 1. (Above left) Normal infant (10 weeks) thymus (25 gm) demonstrating its typical bilobed pyramidal shape. [From Hofmann W, Otto HF. Anatomy and Embryology of the Thymus. In: Walter E, Willich E, Webb WR, eds. The Thymus. Berlin, Heidelberg, New York: Springer-Verlag, 1992.]

Fig. 2. (Above right) Low power view of the normal thymus demonstrating the dense cortical region composed predominantly of thymocytes and the less dense medullary region with Hassel's corpuscles (arrow) and fewer lymphocytes. The fibrous septa subdividing the lobes into lobules extend from the capsule to the corticomedullary junction. [From Hofmann W, Otto HF. Anatomy and Embryology of the Thymus. In: Walter E, Willich E, Webb WR, eds. The Thymus. Berlin, Heidelberg, New York: Springer-Verlag, 1992.]

ARTERIAL BLOOD SUPPLY OF THE THYMUS

Although the arterial blood supply of the thymus originates from all of the neighboring arteries,[9] there are three principle sources. The *posterior thymic arteries* are direct branches of the aorta or of the brachiocephalic artery; generally one artery divides into branches for both lobes and reach their maximal size during childhood.[10] Occasionally they can arise from the middle thyroid artery, the thyrothymic artery.[10] The *superior thymic arteries* usually originate from the inferior thyroid artery but occasionally from the superior thyroid artery.[11,12] *The lateral thymic arteries* are rarely symmetric. In most cases they are branches of the right internal thoracic artery,[7] but sometimes originate from the superior phrenic artery, itself a branch of the internal thoracic artery.

The thymus does not have a distinct hilus or single point of entry or exit for vascular structures. The arteries often enter dorsally through the thymic capsule and course along the connective tissue septa to the corticomedullary junction where they turn to run as arterioles between the cortex and medulla.[2] Siegler[13] reports that the arteries branch, after passing through the capsule, and enter the cortex directly. Capillaries run radially into the cortex and return to the corticomedullary junction, with the medulla receiving irregular branches. According to Williams and Warwick,[12] the thymus contains high-walled postcapillary venules similar to those of the lymph nodes.

The perivascular spaces of the thymus consist of connective tissue regions that are formed when the thymic anlage is invaginated by blood vessels during the seventh gestational week.[8] These spaces are thus continuous with the connective tissue surrounding the gland and each of its lobes. The major components of the perivascular spaces are the blood vessels to and from the medulla. The major arteries rarely branch until they reach the medulla where they run along the corticomedullary junction. Small capillaries entering the cortex may either go straight through to the capsule and leave the gland or loop back in arcades in the deep cortex and/or the outer cortex (close to the subcapsular region).[14,15] Cortical capillaries are all ensheathed by type 1 epithelial cells (subcapsular/perivascular) and normally have a small perivascular space that often contains only collagen and matrix. Blood vessels traversing the cortex differ from those in many other organs by being separated from the cortex by a complete layer of nonendothelial cells. The only other major organ with a similar arrangement is the brain, where astrocytes send pericapillary foot processes to wrap around the blood capillaries thus creating a physiologically important part of the blood-brain barrier. The thymic morphologic arrangement, therefore, seems similar and consistent with the concept of the thymus having a *blood-thymus barrier* which might allow the thymus to exist as an antigenically pure environment. This idea arose from Marshall and White's experiments[16] where germinal centers were only found when antigen was injected directly into the thymus. However, since recent work[17] has shown that self-antigens may enter the thymus through a transcapsular route, the functional significance of this precise perivascular arrangement will require further investigation.

Venous Blood Supply

The thymic veins, which do not run in parallel with the thymic arteries,[9,18] typically consist of large veins following the interlobar septa from the corticomedullary junction to the thymic capsule, as well as small veins that leave the thymic cortex to form venous plexus on the posterior surface of the thymus capsule. The principal thymic veins consist of one or two veins named the thymic posterior vein(s) [the great vein(s) of Keynes][19] which is the fusion of many smaller veins draining the bulk of the caudal aspect of the thymus and empties directly into the inferior left brachiocephalic vein just proximal to the entry of the superior intercostal vein.[6] In approximately fifty percent of humans, there are also superior thymic veins draining the cranial aspect of the thymus and emptying into the inferior thyroid vein (Fig. 3). Accessory thymic veins are rarer and usually drain the lateral aspect of the thymus and empty into the internal mammary veins.[20] Additional veins may drain to the inferior thyroid vein, the thyroidea ima vein and the internal thoracic vein.[6]

Lymphatic Vessels of the Thymus

Consistent with its relatively antigenically protected status, an afferent lymphatic system does not appear to enter the thymus.[6,21,22] The efferent lymphatic drainage of the thymus originates as small lymph capillaries in the perivascular spaces of the medulla or corticomedullary junction.[23] These small lymphatic capillaries subsequently converge within the thymic lobule to form larger vessels that run with the perilobular veins and the thymic venous pedicles to reach the capsule.[24] The lymphatic drainage of the thymus is divided into three groups: the superior lymphatic ducts which drain

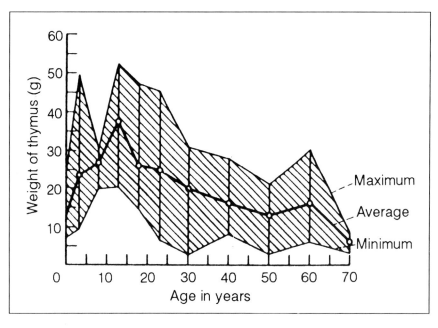

Fig. 3. *Normal weight range of the human thymus during life, according to the findings of Hammar (1926). [From Hofmann W, Otto HF. Anatomy and Embryology of the Thymus. In: Walter E, Willich E, Webb WR, eds. The Thymus. Berlin, Heidelberg, New York: Springer-Verlag, 1992.]*

the superior aspects of the thymus into the internal jugular, brachiocephalic, or anterior mediastinal lymph nodes; the anterior lymphatic ducts which are more numerous and drain the anterior thymus into the parasternal lymph nodes; and the posterior lymphatic ducts which drain the posterior thymus into the tracheobronchial lymph nodes.[6] The efferent lymph vessels or the brachiocephalic nodes unite with efferents from the tracheobronchial nodes to form the left and right bronchomediastinal lymph trunks which most frequently drain independently into the ipsilateral internal jugular and sub-clavian veins. Sometimes, however, the left bronchomediastinal trunk may join the thoracic duct which drains into the left subclavian vein, and the right trunk may join the right lymphatic duct.[12]

INNERVATION OF THE THYMUS

The innervation of the thymus is derived from bilateral branches of the descending vagus, phrenic, hypoglossal, and occasionally the recurrent la-ryngeal nerves.[25] Additionally, the cervicothoracic (stellate, inferior cervical) ganglion and the ansa cervicalis (ansa hypoglossi) have also been described as contributing to the innervation of the thymus. The vagus nerve contains both special visceral (branchial) efferent fibers originating in the nucleus ambiguus and innervate striated (skeletal) muscle, and general visceral (para-sympathetic) efferent fibers originating in the dorsal motor vagus nucleus and serving smooth and cardiac muscle.

It has been demonstrated[26] that the central portion of the thymus an-lage, while still in the neck (middle of second month of gestation) receives branches from both the right and left vagus nerve. These branches enter from the dorsal, lateral, or medial aspect and form a plexus in the medulla. After the organ has descended, it receives sympathetic innervation from ganglia positioned near the thoracic inlet. These fibers, with blood vessels, usually penetrate the investing capsule of the thymus into the substance of the thymus by following the interlobular thymic vasculature.[24] After the differentiation of cortex and medulla, these nerves form varicose plexuses in the subcapsular cortex and at the corticomedullary junction while individual varicose fibers penetrate into the cortex.

There is now good evidence for a noradrenergic network of nerves within the thymus.[27] Since sympathetic stimulation and catecholamines have been shown to promote the exit of cells from the bone marrow, spleen, and lymph nodes, a similar effect has been postulated for the thymus.[25] Catecholamines may influence thymocytes in vivo since developing thymocytes which express β_2-adrenoceptors reduce their proliferation and enhance differentiation marker expression when stimulated in vitro.[28,29] In contrast, thymocyte proliferation is enhanced following chemical sympathectomy at birth with 6-hydroxydopamine (6-OHDA), while there is a decrease in proliferative activity in peripheral lymphocytes.[27,30] Additionally, it has been demonstrated that in the adult rat, 6-OHDA injections caused a highly significant increase in apoptosis and consequent decrease in cortical thymocytes over the eight-day period after sympathectomy, although there was a significant increase in thymocyte proliferation.[31] Studies in animal models have also demonstrated that the aging rodent thymus does not lose its adrenergic innervation,[27] and can be revitalized following hormonal manipulations of the host (see section on involution).[32,33] Future work will be required to determine if similar findings occur in man.

INVOLUTION

Several changes in thymic morphology during aging are known to occur as normal age-dependent thymic involution. Hammer[34,35] initially found an increase in the weight of the thymus until puberty followed by a continuous loss of weight thereafter. Since both the thymus tissue mass and the degree of fatty infiltration within different age groups are quite variable (Fig. 4), attempts were made to further evaluate age-related changes in the thymus. LeBrecque et al[36] demonstrated that thymic tissue that could be reliably evaluated was found at necropsy in 91% of patients ranging in age from 18 to 92 years. Thymic biopsies from 89 patients immediately before thyroidectomy for nontoxic nodular goiter[37] demonstrated that the cortex atrophied slightly faster than the medulla in young people (mean age 17 years), but not in older people (mean age 57 years). Although the numbers of patients in any age category were low and standard deviations were high, there was evidence for an age-related biphasic pattern of cortical involution (but not medulla) in women. This atrophy occurred faster before the fourth decade of life, and thereafter was linear as was found in the male thymus.

The age-dependent weight loss is the result of a progressive loss of lymphatic tissue of both the thymic cortex and medulla, and an accumulation of fat tissue, which has a lower specific gravity than lymphatic tissue, within the perivascular spaces and the thymic septal spaces. These changes begin as early as the first year of life and lead to a nearly complete lipomatous atrophy of the organ in individuals older than 50 years. Although the thymus then consists predominantly of fat tissue in a fibrous capsule with only thin strips of residual lymphatic tissue, it can be detected in vivo radiographically with computed tomography.[38] However, it is now well established that even in those individuals with only remnants of lymphatic tissue, the thymus nevertheless retains the ability to serve its function in cell-mediated immunologic responses by providing new T cells (Leu-6[+] thymocytes, early differentiation marker, CD1a).[39-42]

This normal age-dependent thymic involution may be accelerated under certain circumstances, a fact which becomes especially important in children. This accidental involution of the thymus or thymic atrophy must not be confused with some aspects of thymic dysgenesis. Any kind of stress resulting in elevated blood levels or corticosteroid hormones, corticosteroid therapy, chemotherapy, radiotherapy of the mediastinum, and malnutrition may lead to accidental involution.[43,44] The histologic picture of thymic atrophy in man is similar to that described in animals after the injection of glucocorticosteroids.[45] Necrosis of cortical thymocytes and their resorption by phagocytosing macrophages lead to a drastic reduction of cortical thymocytes without significant modification of the medulla. Thus, a reversal of normal thymic histology is achieved, with a lymphocyte poor cortex and a relatively dense medulla. In addition, Hassel's corpuscles generally persist and become multicystic. The existence of Hassel's corpuscles within the atrophic thymus helps to distinguish between thymic atrophy and thymic dysgenesis where Hassel's corpuscles are not found. The accidental involution of the thymus is reversible,[46] and may even lead to rebound thymic hyperplasia.

While the thymus generally involutes with age, this does not necessarily mean that it becomes nonfunctional. Recent work has shown that while the thymus of aging rats (18 months old) is virtually nonexistent, 30 days after orchiectomy or implantation of a stable analogue of luteinizing hormone-releasing hormone, the thymus reappeared as a large bilobed organ and the peripheral blood lymphocyte counts were dramatically increased.[32] Further experiments have determined that thymic involution is preventable by administering subcutaneous implants of testosterone.[33] If the human thymus is affected in a similar fashion, these findings may be of great importance in the search for methods to boost the body's immune responses, and in efforts to induce thymic tolerance.

The composition of the thymic microenvironment changes with age. Perivascular spaces and connective tissue septae are widening at the expense of the epithelial thymus tissue proper. These areas of reticular connective tissue become filled with adipose tissue so that the grey-pink color of the adolescent thymus changes to white. The involution of the thymus with age is characterized by a puberty-independent continuous degeneration of the thymic epithelial space.[47,48] However, remnants of the thymic epithelial tissue with a cortical lymphocyte population are preserved beyond 100 years of age, and the thymus acts as a site of T lymphocyte differentiation and maturation throughout the whole life of the organism.

References

1. Cardelli NF. Developmental Anatomy and Morphology of the Thymus. In: Cardelli, ed. The thymus in health and senescence. 1st ed. Boca Raton: CRC Press, 1989: 28-29.

2. Kendall MD. Anatomy. In: Givel, ed. Surgery of the thymus. 1st ed. Berlin: SpringerVerlag, 1990: 19-26.

3. Rosai J, Levine GD. Tumors of the Thymus. In: Atlas of Tumor Pathology. Second Series, Fascicle 13. Washington: Armed Forces Institute of Pathology, 1976: 17-26.

4. Otto HF. Pathologie des Thymus. In: Doerr W, Seifert G, Uehlinger E, eds. Spezielle patholoische Anatomic. Vol 17. Berlin: Springer-Verlag, 1984: 43-65.

5. Gilmour JR. Some developmental abnormalities of the thymus and parathyroids. J Pathol Bacteriol 1941; 52: 213-18.

6. Goldstein G, MacKay IR. The human thymus. Lab Invest 1969; 31: 473-87.

7. Gray H. The Lymphatic System. In: Gross, ed. Anatomy of the Human Body. 29th ed. Philadelphia: Lea and Febiger, 1973: 772-73.

8. Norris EH. The morphogenesis and histogenesis of the thymus gland in man, in which the origin of the Hassel's corpuscles of the thymus is discovered. Contrib Embryol 1938; 27: 191-221.

9. Bohm E, Holmgren HJ. Arterial supply of the human thymus. Acta Anat 1946; 2: 98-100.

10. Sarrazin R, Gabelle P, Dyon JF. Anatomical background of the thymus. In: Sarrazin R, Vrousos C, Vincent F, eds. Thymic Tumors. Basel: Karger, 1989: 1-8.

11. Dawson HL. Basic Human Anatomy. New York: Appleton-Century-Crofts, 1966: 148-49.

12. Williams PL, Warwick R, eds. The Lymphatic System. In: Gray's Anatomy. 36th ed. Edinburgh: Churchill-Livingston, 1980; 770, 782-800.

13. Siegler R. The morphology of the thymuses and their relation to leukemia. In: Good RA, Gabrielsen AE, eds. The Thymus in Immunobiology: Structure, Function, and Role in Disease. New York: Hoeber, Harper and Row, 1964: 623.

14. Zaidi SAA. Structure and function of the blood vessels of the thymus. Ph.D. Thesis. London: University of London, 1988: 34-56.

15. Blanc F. Contribution a l'etude de la microvascularisation du lobule thymique chez l'homme. Arch Anat Histol Embryol Norm et Exp 1974; 56: 223-42.

16. Marshall AHE, White RG. The immunological reactivity of the thymus. Br J Exp Pathol 1961; 42: 224-32.

17. Nieuwenhuis P, Stet RJM, Wagebaar JPA et al. The transcapsular route: a new way for (self) antigens to by-pass the blood-thymus barrier. Immunol Today 1988; 9: 372-75.

18. Olivier E, Papamilitiades M. Les veines du thymus. J Anat 1949; 55: 316-19.

19. Last RJ. Anatomy Regional and Applied. 7th ed. Edinburgh: Churchill-Livingston, 1984: 228-29.

20. Hollinshead WH. Anatomy for Surgeons. 2nd ed. (Vol. 2). New York: Harper and Row, 1971: 37-39.

21. Bloodworth JMB Jr., Hiratsuka H, Hickey RC, Wu J. Ultrastructure of the human thymus, thymic tumors, and myasthenia gravis. In: Sommer SC, ed. Pathology Annual. Vol. 10. New York: Appleton-Century-Crofts, 1975: 329-91.

22. Bloodworth JMB Jr., Hiratsuka H, Hickey RC, Wu J. Ultrastructure of the human thymus, thymic tumors, and myasthenia gravis. In: Sommer SC, ed. Pathology Annual. Vol. 10. New York: Appleton-Century-Crofts, 1975: 329-51.

23. Kendall MD. The morphology of perivascular spaces in the thymus. Thymus 1989; 13: 157-64.

24. Aryn S, Gilbert EF, Hong R, Bloodworth JMB Jr. The Thymus. In: Bloodworth JMB Jr., ed. Endocrine Pathology: General and Surgical. 2nd ed. Baltimore: Williams and Wilkins, 1982: 767-832.

25. Kendall MD. Functional anatomy of the thymic microenvironment. J Anat 1991; 177: 1-29.

26. Hammer JA. Konstitutions anatomische studien uber die neurotijierung des menschenembryos. IV. Uber die innervations verhaltnisse der inkretorgane und der thymus bis in den 4. Fotalmonat. 2 Mikrosk Anat Forsch 1935; 38: 53-60.

27. Felten DL, Felten SY. Innervation of the thymus. Thymus Update 1989; 2: 73-88.

28. Singh U, Owen JJT. Studies on the maturation of thymus stem cells—the effects of catecholamines, histamine, and peptide hormones on the expression of T alloantigens. Eur J Immunol 1976; 6: 59-62.

29. Singh U. Effect of catecholamines on lymphopoiesis in fetal mouse explants. J Anat 1979; 129: 279-92.

30. Felten DL, Felten SY, Bellinger DL, et al. Noradrenergic sympathetic neural interactions with the immune system: structure and function. Immunological Reviews 1987; 100: 225-60.

31. Kendall MD, Al-Shawaf A. The innervation of the rat thymus. Brain, Behavior, and Immunity 1991; 5: 9-28.

32. Fitzpatrick FTA, Kendall MD, Wheeler MJ, et al. Reappearance of thymus of aging rats after orchiectomy. J Endocrinol 1985; 106: R17-22.

33. Fitzpatrick TA, Kendall MD, Wheeler MJ, et al. Reappearance of the thymus in aging male rats treated for one month with a stable analogue of luteinizing hormone-releasing hormone J Endocrinol 1986; 108 (Suppl.: Abstract 32).

34. Hammer JA. Uber Gewicht, Involution, und Persistenz des Thymus im Postfotalenben des Menschen. Arch Anat Physiol, Anat Abt 1906; (Suppl) 91: 1982-84.

35. Hammer JA. Der menschenthymus in gesundheit und krankheit: Ergebnisse der numerischen analyse von mehr als tausend menschlichen thymusdrusen. Teil 1: Das normale organ-zugleich eine kritische beleuchtung der Lehre des "Status thymicus." Z Mikrosk Anat Forsch 1926; 6(Suppl): 1-57.

36. LaBrecque PG, Souadjian JV, Titus JL. Etude morphologique quantitative du Thymus human dans une serie d'autopsies. Union Med Can 1972; 101: 695-99.

37. Simpson JG, Gray ES, Beck JS. Age involution in the human adult thymus. Clin Exp Immunol 1975; 19: 261-66.

38. Moore AV, Korobkin M, Olanow W, et al. Age-related changes in the thymus gland. CT-pathologic correlation. Amer J Radiol 1983; 141: 291-94.

39. Stutman O, Good RA. Duration of thymic function. Semin Hematol 1974; 7: 504-23.

40. vonGaudecker B. Ultrastructure of the age-involuted adult human thymus. Cell Tissue Res. 1978; 186: 507-25.

41. Kendall MD. Have we underestimated the importance of the adult human thymus? Experientia 1984; 40: 1181-85.

42. Clark AG, MacLennan KA. The many facets of thymic involution. Immunol Today 1986; 7: 204-05.

43. Dourov N. L'atrophie thymo-lymphatique chez le nourrisson apres traitment prolonge a l'ACTH. Pathol Europ 1970; 5: 216-31.

44. vanBaarlen J, Schuurman HJ, Huber J. Acute thymus involution in infancy and childhood: A reliable marker for duration of acute illness. Hum Pathol 1988; 19: 1155-60.

45. Dourov N. Thymic atrophy and immunodeficiency in malnutrition. In: Muller-Hermelink HK, ed. The Human Thymus. Histopathology and Pathology. Berlin: Springer-Verlag, 1986: 127-50.

46. Henry L. "Accidental" involution of the human thymus. J Pathol Bact 1968; 96: 337-43.

47. Steinman GG. Changes in the human thymus during aging. In: Muller-Hermelink HK, ed. The Human Thymus. Histophysiology and Pathology. Vol. 75. Berlin: Springer, 1986: 43-88.

48. Nakahama M, Mori N, Mori S, et al. Immunohistochemical and histometrical studies of the human thymus with special emphasis on age-related changes in medullary epithelial and dendritic cells. Virchows Arch 1990; 58: 245-51.

CHAPTER 5

THYMIC MICROANATOMY

EPITHELIAL CELLS

Although many workers had characterized thymic epithelial cells (sometimes called epithelial reticular cells) by intracellular tonofilaments and desmosomes and staining with keratin-specific antibodies,[1] Wijngaert et al[2] classified them in the human thymus by their ultrastructural morphology. The thymus anlage in the eighth gestational week contains almost exclusively immature epithelial cells (sometimes with cilia), arranged regularly at its periphery and randomly distributed at the center.[3] At approximately the ninth gestational week hemocytoblasts enter the gland and as the medulla gradually develops, the central cells become more spindle-shaped and the first Hassel's corpuscles appear. Interdigitating reticulum cells are seen at 12 weeks of gestation after mesenchymal septa have begun to invade the cortex. Characteristic differences between the cortical and medullary epithelial cells are established by the 15th gestational week, and the adult organization of the epithelial cells appears between the 16th and 20th gestational weeks.[4] The fully mature thymic microenvironment is composed of diverse epithelial cell types and several cells of mesodermal origin. Gelfand et al[5] initially observed that T lymphocytes need contact with epithelial cells and their products to mature. It is now generally accepted that the epithelial cells are mainly responsible for the creation of the necessary microenvironment and provide the factors that promote sequential intrathymic T lymphocyte differentiation and maturation.[6,7] In electron micrographs four different types of epithelial cells can be recognized in distinct locations in the cortex, and an additional two types in the medulla.[2,8-14] Each epithepial type has a different function in providing the proper environment for T lymphocyte maturation. This classification appears to be true for the thymus glands of all vertebrates. The six cell types were intially described by Wijngaert et al[2] as: type 1 (subcapsular/perivascular); type 2 (cortical) which forms a spectrum of cells in the cortex continuous with types 3 and 4 (electron dense, deep cortical); type 5 (medullary) and type 6 (associated with Hassel's corpuscles). Type 1 and 5 share certain cytological features, type 2 or 3 could also give rise to thymic nurse cells (TNC) which have special characteristics, type 4 cells (electron dense cells) are also found in the medulla and type 5 cells, especially in rodents, are probably composed of several subtypes with different functions.

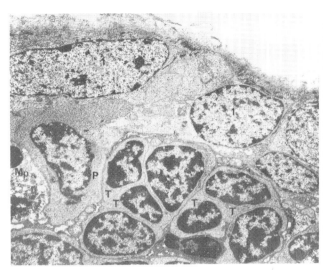

Fig. 1. Type 1 epithelial cells (1) and a probable prothymocyte (P) in the subcapsular zone of the thymus. Type 1 cells form a complete layer under the connective tissue of the capsule. Cortical thymocytes can be seen surrounded by epithelial cell cytoplasm. [From Kendall MD. Histology. In: Givel JC, ed. Surgery of the Thymus. Berlin, Heidelberg, New York: Springer-Verlag, 1990.]

Type 1 epithelial cells, the so-called subcapsular/perivascular epithelium, are an almost uninterrupted layer of cells, joined by desmosomes, which line the surface of the thymus and all perivascular spaces (Fig. 1).[15] These epithelial cells are interposed between stroma, thymic capsule, interlobular septa, and blood vessels of the cortex and corticomedullary junction. Type 1 cells are smaller, contain a large (5-10 µm) heterochromatic nucleus, with a prominent nucleolus, and are more electrondense than those cells which are located somewhat deeper in the cortex. Long strands of rough endoplasmic reticulum are usually present, and the cytoplasm may contain electron-dense granules in addition to the normal organelles. Type 1 epithelial cells may incidentally contain secretory granules and are felt to act as chemoattractants for precursor thymocytes migrating to the thymus.[16]

The surface epithelium forms a flattened sheath that lies on the basal lamina, which separates the thymic epithelial space from the mesenchymal space. It encloses each mesenchymal septum and each perivascular space in the cortex and medulla. Even the smallest capillary is separated by this epithelial cell type from the thymic microenvironment proper. It has been proposed that tight junctions of the cortical capillaries together with perivascular macrophages and the surrounding epithelial cells are the structural basis for the so-called blood-thymus barrier.[17] Thus the thymic cortex has been considered an "antigen-free environment" in which the thymocytes mature. Recently antibody injection studies from Nieuwenhuis et al,[18] however, indicate that antigens can under certain circumstances, in fact, bypass the blood-thymus barrier and enter the cortical region via the transcapsular route. The movement of these molecules is in the same direction as the developing thymocytes, i.e., centripetal. Nieuwenhuis and colleagues argue that this could have important consequences for tolerance induction.[18] The classical blood-thymus barrier apparently does exist, but its functional integrity is not as well defined. Obviously it does not completely sequester cortical maturing T lymphocytes from exposure to self antigens.

Type 2 and 3 epithelial cells predominantly are located in the mid- and outer cortex (Fig. 2). The type 2 cells contain a large (approximately 12 µm)

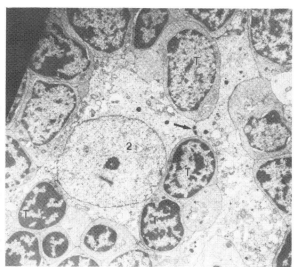

Fig. 2. A type 2 epithelial cell (2) of the thymic cortex. Note the differing morphologies of the cortical thymocytes (T) and the desmosomes between adjacent epithelial cells (arrow). [From Kendall MD. Histology. In: Givel JC, ed. Surgery of the Thymus. Berlin, Heidelberg, New York: Springer-Verlag, 1990.]

leptochromatic (narrow) nucleus and pale-staining cytoplasm containing shorter strands of rough endoplasmic reticulum, than do the type 1 cells, some small, dark inclusions, and occasionally vacuoles. In the fetal thymus it becomes especially clear that cortical thymocytes are frequently embraced by the cytoplasmic processes of these epithelial cells. Type 3 epithelial cells have been defined as "intermediate"[2] and are found mainly in the mid- to deeper cortex and in the medulla. They closely resemble type 2 epithelial cells but contain more vacuoles, a more irregularly shaped nucleus, and electron dense lysosome-like inclusions. It is now thought that the type 2 and 3 cells may represent the in vivo equivalent of the thymic nurse cells, which were first isolated by Wekerle et al.[19] In vitro these thymic nurse cells have the shape of large round lymphoepithelial cell complexes. Their unique characteristic is emperipolesis (lymphocytic penetration of and movement within another cell), a mechanism whereby differentiating thymocytes are enclosed within the thymic nurse cells by an apparently nondestructive process.[20] This creates a unique microenvironment and supports the hypothesis that by internalization thymocytes can be specifically directed in their differentiation and perhaps saved from programmed cell death within the thymus. They have been shown to be binucleated or multinucleated and on average engulf and release 50 to 80 thymic lymphocytes,[21] which functionally and morphologically resemble cortical small thymocytes.

Ritter et al[22] isolated nurse cells from the thymic tissue of human children and demonstrated that in the postnatal thymus, they bear HLA-DR molecules on their surface. HLA-DR molecules are class II antigens of the human major histocompatibility complex (MHC) and are presented to the cortical thymocytes. Some data, especially those of Bevan,[23] Zinkernagel et al,[24] and Zinkernagel[25] indicate that early epithelial contact within the thymic cortex is essential for the MHC-restricted cellular immune reactions and the acquisition of self-tolerance. Wekerle et al[19] speculated that this intimate epithelial contact occurs during the sojourn of cortical thymocytes within thymic nurse cells.

If lymphatic cells in the outer cortical region in situ are enclosed by epithelial cells as seen in vitro after isolation of the thymic nurse cells, this should be obvious in the scanning electron microscope. Therefore, human postnatal thymus obtained from individuals undergoing open heart surgery, or mouse thymus tissue after perfusion fixation with 0.1% glutaraldehyde, were shaken in tissue culture in order to remove free lymphatic cells from the cut surfaces,[10,26] fixed in glutaraldehyde and dried by the critical pont method. Electron microscopy has demonstrated that the outer cortical region epithelial cells, connected to each other by cytoplasmic processes, form large and small aggregates with associated lymphoid cells. Mouse thymic lymphoid cells were observed to migrate into and out of the epithelial lining.[26] There also appears to be cellular communication between these epithelial cells since porcion yellow dye injected into a small number of type 2 and type 3 epithelial cells spreads rapidly throughout the entire thymic cortex.[27,28] This functional syncytium would allow small thymic mitogenic or maturation factors to pass from cell to cell. The epithelium would be able to synchronize a fine control over the number and type of thymocytes produced. It should be noted that since virus particles are smaller than the dye, virus infections could also spread rapidly throughout the thymic lobes.

Type 4 epithelial cells (Fig. 3) are located in the deep cortex and medullary regions of the thymus. They have a heterochromatic, electron-dense irregularly shaped nucleus, and may be binucleated or multinucleated. The dark cytoplasm with long slender processes contains numerous tonofilaments, polyribosomes, swollen mitochondria, numerous vacuoles, and frequently residual bodies or secretory granules. These darkly stained stellate type 4 epithelial cells form a network in the deep thymic cortex and medulla, where they are associated with dark pyknotic thymocytes, or Hassel's corpuscles.

Type 5 epithelial cells (Fig. 4) are undifferentiated and occur in small clusters resting on a basal lamina. They have a round nucleus with some heterochromatin, polyribosomes, and small bundles of tonofilaments and small desmosomes. These cells are primarily found in the corticomedullary region, but also arranged in small groups in the medulla.

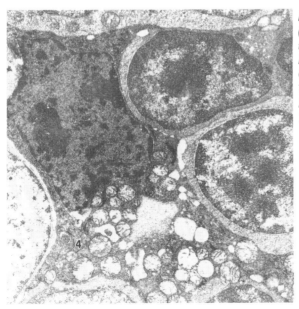

Fig. 3. A type 4 epithelial cell (4) from the deep cortex of the human thymus. [From Kendall MD. Histology. In: Givel JC, ed. Surgery of the Thymus. Berlin, Heidelberg, New York: Springer-Verlag, 1990.]

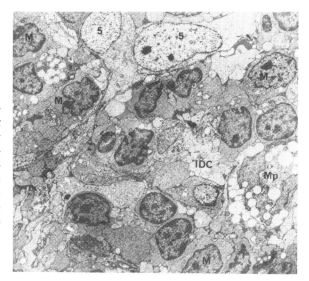

Fig. 4. Type 5 thymic epithelial cells (5) in the thymic medulla. Mp-macrophage; IDC-interdigitating cell cytoplasm. The medullary thymocytes (M) differ from those of the cortex. [From Kendall MD. Histology. In: Givel JC, ed. Surgery of the Thymus. Berlin, Heidelberg, New York: Springer-Verlag, 1990.]

Type 6 "large-medullary" epithelial cells form Hassel's corpuscles in the thymic medulla and are characterized by their large size, abundant tonofilaments, cytoplasmic vesicles with an electron-lucent core and electron-dense halo, and in some cases well-developed, rough endoplasmic reticulum. Norris,[29] who serially sectioned the developing human thymus, proposed that the outer epithelial cell layer in very early stages is derived from the vesicula cervicalis and is, therefore, of ectodermal origin. When the first formation of cortical pseudolobules by mesenchymal septae is most active, some of these ectodermal epithelial cells appear to be separate from the covering epithelial layer and to be displaced into the central region. These separated cells are much larger and of different character than are other central epithelial cells. They can become hypertrophic, synthesize bundles of tonofilaments, and give rise to the Hassel's corpuscles. In the fetus type 6 epithelial cells may be scattered singly, or arranged in small groups.

In fully developed Hassel's corpuscles the cells are concentrically arranged like the lamellae of an onion. These central concentric lamellae lose their nuclei and resemble the horny cells of the epidermis.[30] The morphological similarity to the epidermis suggests an ectodermal origin of the Hassel's corpuscles. This hypothesis is favored by the fact that the corpuscles of Hassel react with anti-epidermal-cell antisera.[31] Functionally, type 6 epithelial cells have been shown to secrete both thymulin and thymosin, factors which induce the differentiation of murine cortical thymocytes, modulate terminal deoxynucleotidyl-transferase (TdT) expression, stimulate lymphocyte mitogen responses, and enhance the production of interferon and macrophage migration inhibitory factor.[32,33]

Hassel's corpuscles are a heterogenous collection of predominately epithelial cells that are a characteristic of the thymic medulla. In their simplest form, they are composed of a few aggregated type 6 cells, but in their larger and more complex form, the epithelial cells exhibit many of the features of keratinized skin[30,34] and contain a variety of cell types (other epithelial cells, eosinophils, macrophages, and occasionally mast cells and plasma cells). Thus, it has been suggested that Hassel's corpuscles are "graveyards" for dead thymocytes and other cell types.[35] It has also been shown that while it is recognized that age, thymic involution and certain diseases can cause Hassel's corpuscles to accumulate antigen,[36] antigenic stimulation can also cause an increase in the number and size of these structures.[37]

Although the epithelial cells are not so phenotypically diverse,[11,38] many differences can be detected with panels of antibodies[39,40] including MHC class II variable expression.[11,41] The MHC antigens are probably made by the epithelial cells[42] and their expression can be induced by cytokines such as γ-interferon (γ-IFN).[43,44] Immunohistochemical staining with anti-HLA-DR (human class II MHC) demonstrates a unique pattern in the postnatal human thymus cortex. In the outer cortex, positively reacting epithelial cell processes surround single or small groups of nonreacting thymocytes. The intimate cell contact seen between cortical thymocytes and epithelial cells resembles the in vitro situation within the thymic nurse cells. In the inner cortex larger areas of tightly packed thymocytes are free of epithelial cells. The lack of contact with nutritive epithelial cells could be a reason for the massive thymocyte cell death in these areas. Steinmann[45] considers this disintegration process to be the beginning of the age-dependent involution which seems to be a continuous physiologic phenomenon. The areas of dying lymphocytes are replaced by widened perivascular spaces which lead to lipomatous atrophy of the thymic cortex. Thus the pattern or extent of MHC class II expression may reflect changes in thymic physiology, and hence could influence the nature of generated thymic subsets.

The origin of these epithelial cells remains unanswered. Norris[29] observed that in 30 mm human embryos, ectodermal cells of the cervical vesicle migrate to completely surround an endodermal thymus primordium. Von Gaudecker and Muller-Hermelink[46] found that the thymus rudiments in 35 mm embryos had two morphologically distinct types of epithelial cells which were sometimes separated from each other: an outer regular row of prismatic cells and an inner mass of polygonal cells. As lymphoid cells infiltrate the thymus, the distinction between different epithelial types becomes difficult but Cordier and Haumont[47] considered that the endoderm of the developing mouse thymus might be invaded by ectoderm, especially in the medulla. Earlier, Norris[29] had also found that as the septa invaded the epithelial primordium, surrounding cells (considered to be ectodermal in origin) broke off and became part of the medulla. Although these observations were based on conventional light microscopy, modern immunocytochemical techniques, using monoclonal antibodies such as A2B5 (which recognizes a complex ganglioside expressed on the cell surface of neurons, neural crest derived cells, and neuropeptide secreting endocrine cells),[48] and various polyclonal antibodies, positively stain the subcapsular/perivascular epithelium and a subpopulation of medullary epithelial cells in the human thymus.[38] These findings indicate that all subcapsular/perivascular and some medullary cells originate from the neural ectoderm. The monoclonal antibodies MR14 and MR19 also react positively with cells around Hassel's corpuscles and cells of the epidermis (ectodermal origin). Hassel's corpuscles and the stratified epithelia of ectodermal origin also have autologous antigens in their intercellular substance[49] and stain positively with antibodies against skin keratins.[50,51]

The relative contributions of both ectodermal and endodermal components to the thymus remain uncertain. At the seventh gestational week, the thymic rudiment, which lacks a medulla, is entirely epithelial and reacts throughout its entirety with the monoclonal antibody A2B5.[52] Only at the 15th gestational week, after lymphoid cells have invaded the organ, is a phenotypically distinct cortex and medulla seen. Based on the induction of MHC antigen expression, Lampert and Ritter[38] postulated that the stem cell is positive for both cortical and subcapsular/medullary markers (a double positive cell). After six to nine days, cultured rat thymic epithelial cells are immunocytochemically positive with both an anticortical and antimedullary antibody and are able to form complete and functional thymus glands when implanted under the kidney capsule of nude rats.[14,53]

The functional importance of these surface markers become apparent in the study of thymomas. Although most are benign and often associated with autoimmune conditions, especially myasthenia gravis, some are clearly malignant.[54] True thymomas are epithelial neoplasms that can support phenotypically normal cortical thymocytes. Those associated with myasthenia gravis (from histologic criteria and single marker studies), were considered to be predominantly of cortical type,[55,56] although they do not express MHC class II antigens. However, thymomas previously considered as cortical with a wide spectrum of thymoma epithelial cell phenotypes are doubly stained when both cortical and subcapsular/medullary markers are used.[9,57] There are very few pure medullary thymomas. Willcox et al[57] examined six invasive thymomas and two pleural thymoma metastases and also found that 50-90% of the epithelial cells were double positive. Lampert and Ritter[38] concluded that the tumorigenic target cell is a double positive stem cell which develops the entire epithelial cell spectrum in the normal thymus. Although the question is still not answered, this stem cell seems to be more likely of endodermal, rather than ectodermal, origin.

This unifying concept of the stem cell's origin of thymic epithelium and its ability to differentiate into other epithelial cell forms could explain some of the pleiomorphic appearances of thymic epithelium. Wijngaert et al[2] noted that the morphologically similar appearance of epithelial cells of the cortex related type 1 cells in the subcapsular/medullary region (including thymic nurse cells) to some of the medullary epithelial cells. Rather than having a separate identity, the double positive stem cell concept suggests that the mature thymic nurse cell could represent the end point of one line of differentiation. By emperipolesis of thymocytes, cortical types 2 or 3 cells could become thymic nurse cells. Simultaneously, genes for the production of molecules that appear in thymic nurse cells but not in most type 2 or 3 cells could be switched on, e.g., by oxytocin and vasopressin which have shown to be important for T-cell subset expansion, differentiation, and maturation.[58]

Other cells of mesodermal origin also contribute to the thymic microenvironment. The interdigitating cells first described in the human thymus by Kaiserling et al[59] in 1974, are probably of monocytogenic origin. In the fetal period, their precursors invade the thymic primordium and settle in the thymic medulla. The fully differentiated interdigitating cell has an irregularly shaped leptochromatic, eccentrically located nucleus with a narrow margin of heterochromatin under the nuclear membrane. The electron lucent cytoplasm of these cells contains centrally-located Golgi membranes, mitochondria, vesicles, and rough endoplasmic reticulum, and extends irregular projections among the epithelial and lymphoid cells on scanning electron microscopy.[26] The interdigitating cells contain characteristic "tennis-racquet-shaped" cytoplasmic inclusions termed Birbeck granules.[60] Unlike the epithelial cells, these cells do not form desmosomes with neighboring cells and their cytoplasm does not contain tonofilaments. Small dark granules and some small phagolysosomes are frequently found in the well developed Golgi. Enclosure by cytoplasmic protrusions of the interdigitating cells allows the microvilli of the medullary thymocytes to interact with the plasmalemma of the interdigitating cells. The significance of this intimate contact is not yet fully understood. It has been suggested that a tubulo-vesicular complex of the interdigitating cells in the medulla and at the corticomedullary junction are an important component of the thymic microenvironment and stimulate T lymphocytes via a humoral signal. They also express the HLA-DR antigens and as antigen presenting cells may contribute to the final maturation of medullary thymocytes. Zinkernagel et al[61] concluded that the murine interdigitating cells have a role in selecting which T-cell precursors are activated to become cytolytic or helper cells during an immunological challenge.

Another cell frequently identified within the human thymus is the myoid cell.[62,63] It is characteristically identified at the corticomedullary junction in the human thymus, close to the capsule, and extending into the medulla. These cells are large single cells, with centrally located indented nuclei and irregularly arranged sarcomeres in the cytoplasm, which may be joined by desmosomes to other (notably epithelial) cells. While myoid cells may have a role in expelling thymocytes from the gland,[64] they have been of primary interest because of their possible role in myasthenia gravis, since Kao and Drachman[65] demonstrated acetylcholine receptors on both myoid and epithelial cells. Although it is known that the thymus is a site of antibody production to acetylcholine receptor substance,[66] the significance of this in the development of myasthenia gravis is not known.

MACROPHAGES

Another important cellular component of the thymic cortical and medullary microenvironment are macrophages,[67] which are considered to play a specific role in T-cell maturation.[68] It is believed that monocytes enter the gland with other circulating stem cells and differentiate either into conventional macrophages which are found at the corticomedullary junction and in the cortex, or into interdigitating cells which typically populate the medulla.[59]

Macrophages have been identified throughout the thymus and in the connective tissues of its capsule and septa. A major role of these cells in the thymus is as potent phagocytes. The greatest numbers are found around the corticomedullary junction, but vary extensively in different patients and probably increase with age. These large cells (15-35 μ in diameter) display all the features of macrophages found elsewhere in the body. A useful identifying feature is that many macrophages have short regions of electron dense plasma membranes that can be seen by electron microscopy. They generally have an irregular and indented nucleus with marginally arranged heterochromatin, but there is variation in the nature and extent of their inclusions.[69] In fetal and neonatal glands, macrophages are potent phagocytes and may contain apoptotic thymocytes and other cellular debris within their cytoplasm. In involuting thymuses, haemotoxylin and eosin staining of these macrophages give a "starry sky" appearance to the cortex. At these times, phagocytosed apoptotic thymocytes and cellular debris are found within the cytoplasm. Rosettes of thymocytes are commonly seen around a central macrophage, e.g., in mouse thymus glands during pregnancy when the glands involute.[70] The formation of tight adhesions with the thymocytes in macrophage rosettes signals changes in thymocyte membranes that occur with the initiation of apoptosis.[71]

Athough most macrophages usually contain a range of phagosome-like inclusions, there are times when they are not very active. Other functions of macrophages then become dominant, depending on the physiology of other cells in the local environment. These functions include cytokine production and release[72] which probably affect all stages of thymocyte proliferation, maturation, and differentiation and thymocyte ontogeny, since it is known that macrophages produce and express receptors for many different cytokines, e.g., IL-1, IL-2, IL-4, IL-6, IL-10, tumor necrosis factor α and γ-interferon. Additionally, macrophages secrete a mitogenic thymocyte-differentiating factor[73] which induces the functional maturation of thymocytes in vitro and possibly in vivo.[74]

Beller et al[75] found that approximately 75% of thymic macrophages are HLA-DR positive and are very effective in antigen presentation to T lymphocytes in vitro, and therefore, function as central cells in an immune response. MHC class II positive macrophages take up, process and present antigen in conjunction with a surface MHC molecule, to T lymphocytes, particularly CD4+ cells which are activated to proliferate (often through the release of IL-1). In the thymic cortex, MHC class II positive thymic interdigitating cells probably function as antigen presenting cells.[76] Hamblin and Edgeworth concluded that tolerance induction to self-MHC and self MHC restriction are more likely to be the function of these MHC class II positive cells. Indeed, negative selection of differentiating thymocytes through these cells can result in tolerance.[12]

MYOID CELL

Another cell type, probably derived from the mesoderm, is the large myoid cell. These cells are a regular feature of the human thymus and are unevenly distributed throughout the gland, frequently grouped in clusters at the corticomedullary junction that extend into the medulla. In contrast to epithelial cells, these large rounded or elongated cells, with centrally located indented nuclei and irregularly arranged sarcomeres in the cytoplasm, exhibit a strong immunoreactivity with anti-striated muscle myosin, but not with the antibody to smooth muscle myosin.[78] Ultrastructurally myoid cells resemble degenerating striated muscle. Rounded myoid cells (up to 40 μm in diameter) are preponderant in both children and adults. They generally possess a centrally or eccentrically located single nucleus and large amounts of randomly oriented myofilaments. Often they are arranged in concentric bundles or intertwined in vortices and are frequently joined by desmosomes to other (notably epithelial) cells. In the elongated or spindle-shaped myoid cells, myofilaments are roughly oriented along the main axis of the cell.[79]

However, a precise alignment of thin and thick filaments, giving rise to regular sarcomeres is infrequently found within these cells. The function of these myoid cells in the normal thymus is obscure. It has been suggested that myoid cells may play a critical role in the pathogenesis of the autoimmune disease myasthenia gravis,[80] since it has been demonstrated[65] that acetylcholine receptors are on myoid (and epithelial) cells. In myasthenia gravis, antibodies produced in the thymus to the acetylcholine receptor circulate in the serum.[66,81]

T LYMPHOCYTES

In the adult thymus, vessels at the corticomedullary junction appear to be the site of incoming hematopoietic T lymphocyte precursors. The thymocytes of the adult human thymus are generally small cells with a pachychromatic nucleus and few cytoplasmic organelles. However, detailed ultrastructural studies have demonstrated a large range of cellular morphology among thymocytes.[82] Incoming thymocytes appear first in association with Ia negative macrophages, in the border region of the cortex and the medulla, and two to three days later can also be found aggregating with the Ia positive medullary interdigitating dendritic cells and with a population of epithelial thymic nurse cells in the subcapsular cortex (Fig. 5).[19,83-85] Lymphoepithelial complexes have been described in which the thymocytes are enclosed in plasma membrane vesicles or infoldings[18] of fluorescent staining thymic nurse cells.[86,87] A distinctive thymocyte population in the outer cortex that associates with thymic nurse cells are commonly in mitosis. These large (9-14 µm), contain self-renewing thymocytes make up between 5 and 15% of the total thymocyte population and give rise to three other populations: the deep cortical small thymocytes, the juxtamedullary and medullary midsize thymocytes, and the thymic cell emigrants.[88,89] These heterogenous outer cortical thymocytes are themselves apparently derived from the thymus homing precursors after a significant lag period. The range of morphology observed in cells of this zone (Fig. 6) reflects cells passing through the mitotic cycle.

Three major types of thymocytes in the outer thymic cortex are further identified by surface markers: CD4⁻8⁻3⁻ (double negative) cells, CD4⁻8⁺3⁻ cells, and CD4⁺8⁺3⁻/lo (double positive) cells.[90,91] The CD3⁻ (and, therefore, T-cell receptor [TCR] negative) double negative cells appear to be the most primitive progenitors.[92-96] Experiments involving intrathymic transfer demonstrate that they both proliferate and rapidly give rise first to CD4⁻8⁺TCR⁻/lo cells[92] and then other thymocyte subsets.[93-96] Isolated CD4⁻8⁺TCR⁻/lo outer cortical thymocytes give rise to double positive TCR⁻/lo within one to two cell cycles in vitro[17] or when placed into either irradiated[98] or unirradiated, congenic host thymuses.[99] These double positive TCR⁻/lo cells then give rise to either CD4⁺8⁻ and CD4⁻8⁺ cells[98,99] which express high levels of TCR molecules.[99] The subset of double positive TCR^lo outer cortical thymocytes undergo further positive and/or negative thymic selection to establish self-MHC restriction[100-103] or self-tolerance. Their progeny include numerous deep cortical small double positive TCR^lo cells that are destined to ultimately undergo apoptosis intrathymically,[90,99] while the single positive (CD8 only or CD4 only) TCR^hi cells mature in the juxtamedullary cortex and medulla. A schematic for thymocyte maturation is shown in Figures 5 and 6. Although the lineages shown are likely to be correct, a detailed analysis of cell division, cycle time, self-renewal capacity, number of cell divisions within a phenotypically defined subset, and the proportion of daughter cells that undergo the maturational step from precursor to progeny has not yet been established.

The two major classes of cells in the deep cortex are small double positive TCR^{lo} thymocytes and dendritic cortical epithelial cells. These small double positive TCR^{lo} thymocytes possess scant cytoplasm, make up approximately 85% of the total thymocyte population, share with outer cortical thymocytes a high degree of cortisone sensitivity in vivo, and usually

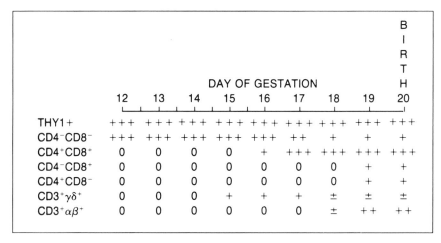

	12	13	14	15	16	17	18	19	20
THY1+	+++	+++	+++	+++	+++	+++	+++	+++	+++
CD4$^-$CD8$^-$	+++	+++	+++	+++	+++	++	+	+	+
CD4$^+$CD8$^+$	0	0	0	0	+	+++	+++	+++	+++
CD4$^-$CD8$^+$	0	0	0	0	0	0	0	+	+
CD4$^+$CD8$^-$	0	0	0	0	0	0	0	+	+
CD3$^+$γδ$^+$	0	0	0	+	+	+	±	±	±
CD3$^+$αβ$^+$	0	0	0	0	0	0	±	++	++

(DAY OF GESTATION, columns 12–20; column 20 labeled BIRTH)

Fig. 5. Development of T cells in the fetal mouse thymus from day 12 to day 20 of gestation. 0, ±, +, ++, +++, refer to the relative abundance of cells having the indicated markers. [From: Raulet DH, Eisen HN. Cellular Basis for Immune Responses. In: Eisen HN, ed. General Immunology, 2nd ed., Philadelphia, J.B. Lippincott, 1990: 104.]

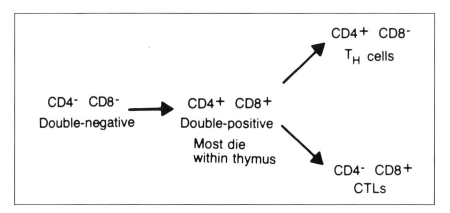

Fig. 6. Schematic of thymocyte maturation within the thymus. Double-negative thymocytes are the progenitors of both double-positive thymocytes and mature T cells. Although double-positive thymocytes are intermediates in thymocyte differentiation, most undergo apoptosis in the thymus. [From: Raulet DH, Eisen HN. Cellular Basis for Immune Responses. In: Eisen HN, ed. General Immunology, 2nd ed., Philadelphia, J.B. Lippincott, 1990: 104.]

die in situ within hours to days. Why and how these cells die is unknown. The deep cortical small thymocytes synthesize high concentrations of terminal deoxynucleotidyl transferase (TdT),[104] which almost certainly plays a major role in generating TCR functional diversity by adding nucleotides to V-D and D-T joints, and contributes to intrathymic apoptosis or death.[105] It has also been proposed that thymocyte death might result from their peculiarly high sensitivity to endogenously produced glucocorticoids[88,106,107] which could result in the characteristic chromatin fragmentation.[108,109]

Most deep cortical thymocytes are peanut agglutinin (PNA) positive,[110] and lack terminal sialic acids on many of their glycolipid and glycoprotein carbohydrate side chains.[111] There appears to be an inverse correlation between the presence of homing receptors (that enable lymphocytes to migrate to particular lymphoid organs) and the presence of surface PNA binding sites. Terminal sialiation could release formerly PNA positive thymocytes from hypothetical PNA-like lectins thus allowing their exit from the thymus.

The deep cortical thymocytes appear to be connected with cortical dendritic epithelial cells, which have long branching dendritic processes from desmosomal junctions.[112] The long axes of these dendritic processes run perpendicular to the corticomedullary junction and the capsule to form lacy vertical networks among interspersed thymocytes. The dendritic cortical epithelial cells are unusual in that they express extremely high levels of class II MHC (Ia antigen) allotypic and monomorphic determinants.[113,114] Immunoelectron microscopic analysis reveals that many of the thymocytes adherent to the dendritic cortical epithelial cells express TCR molecules and bind the Ia antigen of the dendritic cortical epithelial cells.[114] Surprisingly, these dendritic cortical epithelial cells do not express detectable levels of class I MHC allotypic determinants.[115] Thus, the deep cortex of the thymus is dominated by populations of thymocytes that (a) contain a high proportion of cells destined to die, yet (b) give rise to a (major) portion of the thymic emigrant pool, and (c) while in the thymus interact with a defined class of thymic cortical epithelial cells selectively expressing MHC class II antigens.

The juxtamedullary portion of the deep thymic cortex contains, in addition to the double positive small thymocytes and dendritic cortical epithelial cells, increased numbers of mature phenotype (CD3+, TCRhi, single CD4 or CD8 positive) midsized cells.[116] In mice, high levels of both the lymph node (MEL-14) and the Peyer's patch (LPAM-1) homing receptors that can be detected on these cells by both monoclonal and polyclonal rat antibodies.[116] Surprisingly, mature phenotype cells in the adjacent medulla are MEL-14 negative but appear to express high levels of the LPAM-1 α4 chain epitope. Most deep cortical double negative and double positive immature cells express only low levels of these homing receptor antigens. Thus the mature cortical progeny of thymus cell maturation are PNA- and homing receptor positive (HRhi), perhaps reflecting their conditioning for thymic exit to peripheral lymphoid organs. In contrast, their immature double positive cortical associates are PNA+ and HRlo, possibly reflecting their likelihood of intrathymic death.

Recently produced thymocytes migrate from the cortex toward the medulla and stream between the lacy networks formed by the dendritic cortical epithelial cells and the cortical macrophages. On the medullary side of the cortex-medulla junction, macrophages, eosinophils, bone-marrow derived dendritic cells in conjunction with medullary epithelial cells, and occasionally mast cells and plasma cells give rise to Hassel's corpuscles,[112] which have been proposed to be a graveyard for dying thymocytes.[35]

Approximately 10-15% of the CD4+8-TCR[hi] or CD4-8+TCR[hi] medullary thymocytes express high levels of the chain (α4) of the Peyer's patch homing receptor (LPAM-1) but no detectable MEL-14 epitopes. Attempts to demonstrate that cortisone-resistant, mature phenotype medullary cells migrate to the periphery have not succeeded.[107] Thus one must entertain the possibility that at least some of these thymocytes may never emigrate from the thymus or that the emigration process is cortisone sensitive. It is conceivable that some of these thymocytes are retained within the thymus for regulatory and/or developmental functions or represent a potentially dangerous population of self-reactive thymocytes.

It is interesting to note that mature medullary T lymphocytes may be derived by intrathymic maturation or accumulate slowly from a subset of circulating mature (and perhaps antigen-activated) T lymphocytes.[117-120] The relative proportion of medullary thymocytes originating from intrathymic versus extrathymic sources is not known. Extrathymic medullary T lymphocytes may function in the induction of self-tolerance.[120]

The medullary thymocytes are associated with epithelial cells expressing MHC class I determinants. The medulla also contains bone marrow derived MHC class I and class II positive[42,121] interdigitating cells capable of in vitro efficient antigen presentation. The role of these various medullary nonlymphoid cells in the physiology of the thymus and the maturation of thymocytes is unclear, as is the true fate and function of the medullary thymocytes. It is conceivable that the medullary dendritic antigen presenting cells are involved in negative selection of mature intrathymic T lymphocytes bearing high-affinity anti-self T-cell receptors.[100,113]

Small numbers of B lymphocytes are also found in the thymus, even to the extent that follicular structures have been described in the human adult thymus. In the connective tissue, septae and perivascular spaces, different numbers of plasma cells, mast cells and cell types of the myeloid lineage can also be recognized.

In summary, the thymic cortex and/or a subpopulation of the medullary cells give rise to those thymus cell emigrants endowed with all the properties of antigen recognition, cell interaction receptors, and the major immune properties of T lymphocytes.

REFERENCES

1. DeMaagd RA, Mackenzie WA, Schuurman HJ, et al. The human thymus microenvironment: Heterogeneity detected by monoclonal anti-epithelial cell antibodies. Immunology 1985; 54: 745-54.

2. Wijngaert FP van de, Kendall MD, Schuurman HJ, et al. Heterogeneity of human thymic epithelial cells at the ultrastructural level. Cell Tissue Res 1984; 237: 227-37.

3. von Gaudecker B, Muller-Hermelink HK. Ontogenetic differentiation of epithelial and nonepithelial cells in the human thymus. Adv Exp Med Biol 1979;114: 19-23.

4. Muller-Hermelink HK, Steinmann GG. Age-related alterations of intrathymic microenvironments. In: deWeck AL, ed. Lymphoid Cell Functions in Aging.

Topics in Aging Research in Europe. Vol. 3. The Netherlands: Eurage, 1984: 75-82.

5. Gelfand EW, Dosch HM, Shore A, et al. Role of the thymus in human T-cell differentiation. In: Gelfand EW, Dosch HM, eds. Biological Basis of Immunodeficiency. New York: Raven, 1980: 39-66.

6. Steinmann GG, Muller-Hermelink HK. Lymphocyte differentiation and its microenvironment in the human thymus during aging. Monogr Dev Biol 1984; 17: 142-55.

7. Schuurman HJ, Kater L. Relevance of "nurse cells" in histophysiology of lymphoid tissues. Thymus 1985; 7: 13-23.

8. Haynes BF. The human thymic microenvironment. Adv Immunol 1984; 36: 87-142.

9. Maagd RA de, Mackenzie WA, Schuurman HJ, et al. The human thymus microenvironment: Heterogeneity detected by monoclonal anti-epithelial antibodies. Immunology 1985; 54: 745-54.

10. von Gaudecker B. The development of the human thymus microenvironment. In: MullerHermelink HK, ed. The Human Thymus. Histopathology and Pathology. Curr Top Pathol 75. New York: Springer, 1986: 1-41.

11. von Gaudecker B, Steinmann GG, Hansmann ML, et al. Immunohistochemical characterization of the thymic microenvironment. Cell Tissue Res 1986; 244: 403-12.

12. von Gaudecker B, Larche M, Schuurman HJ, et al. Analysis of the fine distribution of thymic epithelial microenvironment molecules by immuno-electron microscopy. Thymus 1989; 13: 187-94.

13. Kendall MD. Anatomical and physiological factors influencing the thymic microenvironment. In: Kendall MD, Ritter MA, eds. Thymus Update. Vol. 1. New York: Harwood Academic Publishers, 1988: 27-65.

14. Kendall MD, Schuurman HJ, Fenton J, et al. Implantation of cocultured thymic fragments in congenitally athymic (nude) rats. Ultrastructural characteristics of the developing microenvironment. Cell Tissue Res 1988; 254: 283-94.

15. von Gaudecker B. Functional histology of the human thymus. Anat Embryol 1991; 183: 1-15.

16. Le Douarin NM, Jotereau FV. The ontogeny of the thymus. In: Kendall MD, ed. The Thymus Gland. London: Academic Press, 1981: 37-62.

17. Raviola E, Karnovsky MJ. Evidence for a blood-thymus barrier using electron-opaque tracers. J Exp Med 1972; 129: 431-42.

18. Nieuwenhuis P, Stet RJM, Wagenaar JPA, et al. The transcapsular route: A new way for (self) antigens to by-pass the blood-thymus barrier? Immunology Today 1988; 9: 372-75.

19. Wekerle H, Ketelsen UP, Ernst M. Thymic nurse cells—lymphoepithelial cell complexes in murine thymuses: morphological and serological characterization. J Exp Med 1980; 151: 925-44.

20. Trowell OA. Intracellular lymphocytes in thymus reticular cells and in fibroblasts cultured in vitro. J Physiol (Lond) 1949; 110: 5P.

21. Scollay R, Andrews P, Boyd R, et al. The role of the thymic cortex and medulla in T-cell differentiation. In: Klaus GGB, ed. Microenvironments in the Lymphoid System. Adv Exp Med Biol 1985; 186: 229-34.

22. Ritter MA, Sauvage CA, Cotmore SF. The human thymus microenvironment in vitro identification of the thymic nurse cell and other antigenetically-

distinct subpopulations of epithelial cells. Immunology 1981; 44: 439-46.

23. Bevan MJ. In a radiation chimera host H-2 antigens determine the immune responsiveness of donor cytolytic cells. Nature 1977; 269: 417-18.

24. Zinkernagel RM, Callahan GN, Althage A, et al. On the thymus in the differentiation of "H-2 self-recognition" by T cells: Evidence for dual recognition? J Exp Med 1978; 147: 882-86.

25. Zinkernagel RM. The thymus: Its influence on recognition of self major histocompatibility antigens by T cells and consequences for reconstitution of immuno deficiency. In: Cooper MD, Lawton AR, Milscher PA, Meuller-Eberhard HJ, eds. Immunodeficiency. Berlin: Springer, 1979: 171-81.

26. van Ewijk W. Cell-surface topography of thymic microenvironments. Lab Invest 1988; 59: 579-90.

27. Kendall MD. The outer and inner thymus cortex is a functional syncytium. Cell Biol Int Rep 1985; 9: 3-9.

28. Kendall MD. The syncytial nature of epithelial cells in the thymic cortex. J Anat 1986; 147: 3-12.

29. Norris EH. The morphogenesis and histogenesis of the thymus gland in man: in which the origin of the Hassel's corpuscles of the human thymus is discovered. Contrib Embryol 1938; 166: 191-221.

30. von Gaudecker B, Scmale EM. Similarities between Hassel's corpuscles of the human thymus and the epidermis. An investigation by electron microscopy and histochemistry. Cell Tissue Res 1974; 151: 347-68.

31. Didierjean L, Saurat JH. Epidermis and Thymus. Similar antigenic properties in Hassel's corpuscle and subsets of keratinocytes. Clin Exp Dermatol 1980; 5: 395-04.

32. Hirokawa K, McClure JE, Goldstein AL. Age-related changes in localization of thymosin in the human thymus. Thymus 1982; 4: 19-29.

33. Schuurman HJ, van de Wijngaert FP, Delvoye L, et al. Heterogenicity and age-dependency of human thymus reticulo-epithelium in production of thymosin components. Thymus 1985; 7: 13-23.

34. Mandel T. The development and structure of Hassel's corpuscles in the guinea pig: A light and electron microscopic study. Z Zellforsch Mikrosk Anat 1968; 89: 180-92.

35. Blau JN. The dynamic behavior of Hassel's corpuscles and the transport of particular matter in the thymus of the guinea pig. Immunology 1967; 13: 281-92.

36. Marshall AHE, White RG. The immunological reactivity of the thymus. Br J Exp Pathol 1961; 42: 379-85.

37. Kater L. A note on Hassel's corpuscles. In: Davies AJS, Carter RL, eds. Contemporary Topics in Immunology. Volume 2. Thymus Dependency. London: Plenum, 1973: 101-09.

38. Lampert IR, Ritter MA. The origin of the diverse epithelial cells of the thymus: Is there a common stem cell? Thymus Update 1988; 2: 5-25.

39. Kampinga J, Berges S, Boyd RL, et al. Thymic epithelial antibodies: immunohistochemical analysis and introduction of nomenclature. Summary of the Epithelium Workshop held at the 2nd Workshop "The Thymus. Histophysiology and Dynamics in the Immune System". Thymus 1989; 13: 165-73.

40. Brekelmans P, van Ewijk W. Phenotypic characterization of murine thymic microenvironments. Seminars in Immunology 1990; 2: 13-24.

41. Bofill M, Janossy G, Willcox N, et al. Microenvironments in the normal and myasthenia gravis thymus. Amer J Pathol 1985; 119: 462-73.

42. Rouse RV, Ezine S, Weissman IL. Expression of major histocompatibility complex antigens in the thymuses of chimeric mice. Transplantation 1985; 40: 422-27.

43. Berrih S, Arenzana F, Cohen S, et al. Interferon-g modulates HLA class II antigen expression on cultured human thymic epithelial cells. J Immunol 1985; 135: 1165-71.

44. Rocha B, Leheun A, Papiernik M. IL-2 dependent proliferation of thymic accessory cells. J Immunol 1988; 140: 1076-80.

45. Steinmann GG. Changes of the human thymus during aging. In: Muller-Hermelink HK, ed. The Human Thymus. Histophysiology and Pathology. Curr Top Pathol. Vol 75. New York: Springer, 1986: 43-88.

46. Gaudecker von B, Muller-Hermelink HK. Ontogeny and organization of the stationary nonlymphoid cells in the human thymus. Cell Tissue Res 1980; 207: 287-306.

47. Cordier AC, Haumont SA. Development of the thymus, parathyroids and ultimobranchial bodies in NMRI and nude mice. Amer J Anat 1980; 157: 191-204.

48. Haynes BF, Shimizu K, Eisenbarth GS. Identification of human and rodent thymus epithelium using tetanus toxin and monoclonal antibody A2B5. J Clin Invest 1983; 71: 9-14.

49. Beletskaya LV, Gnesditskaya EV. Detection of squamous epithelial intercellular substance antigen(s) in Hassel's corpuscles of human and animal thymus. Scand J Immunol 1980; 12: 93-98.

50. Gnesditskaya E, Beletskaya LV. Immunofluorescence study of keratin of Hassel's corpuscles and epidermis of the human skin. Bull Exp Biol Med 1974; 77: 431-33.

51. Takigawa M, Imamura S, Ofuji S. Demonstration of epidermis-specific heteroantigens in thymic epithelial cell. Intern Arch Allergy Appl Immunol 1977; 55: 58-60.

52. Haynes BF, Scearce RM, Lobach DF, et al. Phenotypic characterization and ontogeny of mesodermal derived and endocrine epithelial components of the human thymic microenvironment. J Exp Med 1984; 159: 1149-68.

53. Schuurmann HJ, Vos JG, Broekhuisen R, et al. In vivo biological effect of allogeneic cultured thymic epithelium on thymus dependent immunity in athymic nude rats. Scand J Immunol 1985; 21: 21-30.

54. Rosai J, Levine G. Tumors of the Thymus. Fascicle 13. Washington: Armed Forces Institute of Pathology, 1976.

55. Chilosi M, Iannucci A, Fiore-Donati L, et al. Myasthenia gravis: immunohistological heterogeneity in microenvironmental organization of hyperplastic and neoplastic thymuses suggesting different mechanisms of tolerance breakdown. J Neuroimmunology 1986; 11: 191-204.

56. Muller-Hermelink HK, Marino M, Palestro G. Pathology of the thymic epithelial tumors. In: Muller-Hermelink HK, ed. The Human Thymus. Histopathology and Pathology. Curr Top Path Vol. 75. New York: Springer, 1986: 207-68.

57. Willcox N, Schleup M, Ritter MA, et al. Myasthenic and nonmyasthenic thymoma. An expansion of a minor cortical epithelial subset? Amer J Path 1987; 127: 447-60.

58. Geenen V, Defresne MP, Robert F, et al. The neurohormonal thymic microenvironment: Immunocytochemical evidence that thymic nurse cells are neuroendocrine cells. Neuroendocrinology 1988; 47: 365-68.

59. Kaiserling E, Stein H, Muller-Hermelink HR. Interdigitating reticulum cells in the human thymus. Cell Tissue Res 1974; 155: 47-55.

60. Birbeck MS, Breathnach AS, Everall JD. An electron microscope study of basal melanocytes and high-level clear cells (Langerhans cells) in vitiligo. J Invest Dermatol 1961; 37: 51-64.

61. Zinkernagel RM, Callahan GN, Althage A, Cooper S, Klein PA, Klein J. On the thymus in the differentiation of "H-2 self-recognition" by T cells: Evidence for dual recognition? J Exp Med 1978; 147: 882-96.

62. Henry K. An unusual thymic tumor with a striated muscle (myoid) component. Br J Dis Chest 1972; 66: 291-99.

63. Bockman DE, Winborn WB. Ultrastructure of thymic myoid cells. J Morphol 1969; 129: 201-10.

64. Henry K. The human thymus in disease with particular emphasis on thymitis and thymoma. In: Kendall MD, ed. The Thymus Gland. London: Academic Press, 1981: 85-111.

65. Kao I, Drachman DB. Thymic muscle cells bear acetylcholine receptors: Possible relation to myasthenia gravis. Science 1977; 195: 74-75.

66. Vincent A, Scadding GK, Thomas HL, Newsom-Davis J. In vitro synthesis of anti-acetylcholine-receptor antibody by thymic lymphocytes in myasthenia gravis. Lancet 1: 305-07.

67. Duijvestijn AM, Hoefsmit ECM. Ultrastructure of the rat thymus: The microenvironment of T lymphocyte maturation. Cell Tissue Res 1981; 218: 279-92.

68. Beller DI, Unanue ER. Ia antigens and antigen-presenting function of thymic macrophages. J Immunol 1980; 124: 1433-40.

69. Kendall MD. Histology. In: Givel JC, ed. Surgery of the Thymus. New York: Springer-Verlag, 1990: 33-38.

70. Clarke A, Kendall MD. Histological changes in the mouse thymus during pregnancy. Thymus 1990; 14: 65-78.

71. Kendall MD. The cell biology of cell death in the thymus. Thymus Update 1990; 3: 47-70.

72. Kendall MD. Functional anatomy of the thymic microenvironment. J Anat 1991; 177: 1-29.

73. Beller DI, Unanue ER. Thymic maturation in vitro by a secretory product from macrophages. J Immunol 1977; 118: 1780-87.

74. Beller DI, Farr AG, Unanue ER. Regulation of lymphocyte proliferation and differentiation by macrophages. Fed Proc 1978; 37: 91-96.

75. Beller Dl, Unanue ER. Evidence that thymocyte require at least two distinct signals to proliferate. J Immunol 1979; 123: 2890-93.

76. Hamblin AS, Edgeworth JD. Does antigen presentation occur in the thymus? Thymus Update 1988; 1: 135-53.

77. Kyewski BA, Fathman CG, Rouse RV. Intrathymic presentation of circulating non-MHC antigens by medullary dendritic cells: An antigen-dependent microenvironment for T-cell differentiation. J Exp Med 1986; 163: 231-46.

78. Drenckhahn D, von Gaudecker B, Muller-Hermelink HK, et al. Myosin- and actin-containing cells in the human postnatal thymus. Ultrastructural and immunohistochemical findings in normal thymus and in Myasthenia Gravis. Virchows Arch 1979; 32: 3345-50.

79. Gaudecker B von. Functional histology of the human thymus. Anat Embryol 1991; 183: 1-15.

80. Wekerle H, Muller-Hermelink HK. The Thymus in Myasthenia Gravis. In: Muller-Hermelink HK, ed. The Human Thymus, Histophysiology and Pa-

thology. Curr Top Pathol 75. New York/: Springer, 1986: 179-206.

81. Lindstrom J. Autoimmune response to acetylcholine receptor in myasthenia gravis and its animal model. Adv Immunol 1979; 27: 1-50.

82. VonGaudecker B. Ultrastructure of the age-involuted adult human thymus. Cell Tissue Res 1978; 186: 507-25.

83. Fink PJ, Weissman IL, Kaplan HS, et al. The immunocompetence of murine stromal cell associated thymocytes. J Immunol 1984; 132: 2266-72.

84. Boniver J, Houben-Defresne MP, Varlet A, et al. "Thymic nurse cells" contain the first virus-producing cells after radiation leukemia virus inoculation in C57BL/Ka mice. Adv Exp Med Biol 1982; 149: 263-68.

85. Kyewski BA, Rouse RV, Kaplan HS. Thymocyte rosettes: Multicellular complexes of lymphocytes and bone marrow-derived stromal cells in the mouse thymus. Proc Natl Acad Sci USA 1982; 79: 5646-51.

86. Scollay R, Weisman IL. Thymocyte and thymus migrant subpopulations defined with monoclonal antibodies to the antigens Lyt-1, Lyt-2 and ThB. J Immunol 1980; 124: 2841-45.

87. Scollay R, Jacobs S, Jerabek L, et al. T-cell maturation: Thymocyte and thymus migrant subpopulations defined with monoclonal antibodies to MHC region antigens. J. Immunol. 1980; 124: 2845-50.

88. Weissman IL. Thymus cell maturation: Studies on the origin of cortisone-resistant thymic lymphocytes. J Exp Med 1973; 137: 504-09.

89. Fathman CG, Small M, Herzenberg LA, et al. Thymus cell maturation . II. Differentiation of three "mature" subclasses in vivo. Cell Immunol 1975; 15: 109-14.

90. Scollay R, Butcher E, Weissman IL. Thymus cell migration. Quantitative aspects of cellular traffic from the thymus to the periphery in mice. Eur J Immunol 1980; 10: 210-18.

91. Guidos C, Weissman IL, Adkins B. Intrathymic injection of fetal and adult CD4-8-thymocytes: Analysis of thymic and peripheral progeny. J Immunol 1988; 136: 678-82.

92. Adkins B, Miller C, Okada CY, et al. Early events in T-cell maturation. Annu Rev Immunol 1987; 5: 325-78.

93. Scollay R, Wilson A, D'Amico A, et al. Development status and reconstitution potential of subpopulations of murine thymocytes. Immunol Rev 1980; 104: 81-93.

94. Fowlkes BJ, Pardoll DM. Molecular and cellular events of T-cell development. Adv Immunol 1989; 12: 1-23.

95. Crispe IN, Moore MW, Husmann LA, et al. Differentiation potential of subsets of CD4-8-thymocytes. Nature 1987; 329: 336-39.

96. Kingston R, Jenkinson EJ, Owen JJT. A single stem cell can recolonize an embryonic thymus, producing phenotypically distinct T-cell populations. Nature 1985; 317: 811-13.

97. Paterson DJ, Williams AF. An intermediate cell in thymocyte differentiation that expresses CD8 but not CD4 antigen. J Exp Med 1987; 166: 1603-13.

98. Kikolic-Zugic J, Bevan MJ. Thymocytes expressing CD8 differentiate into CD4+ cells following intrathymic injection. Proc Natl Acad Sci USA 1988; 85: 8633-38.

99. Guidos CJ, Weissman IL, Adkins B. Intrathymic maturation of murine T lymphocytes. J Immunol 1989; 143: 1003-09.

100. Kappler JW, Wade T, White J, et al. A T-cell receptor Vβ segment that imparts reactivity to a class II major histocompatibility complex product. Cell

1987; 49: 273-79.

101. Kisielow P, Bluthman L, Staerz UD, et al. Tolerance in T-cell receptor transgenic mice involves deletion of nonmature CD4$^+$ 8$^+$ thymocytes. Nature 1988; 333: 742-45.

102. MacDonald HR, Hergartner H, Pedrazzini T. Intrathymic deletion of self-reactive cells prevented by neonatal anti-CD4 antibody treatment. Nature 1988; 335: 174-77.

103. Fowlkes BJ, Schwartz RH, Purdoll NM. Deletion of self-reactive thymocytes occurs at the CD4$^+$8$^+$ precursor stage. Nature 1988; 334: 620-22.

104. Kincade PW, Lee G, Pietrangeli CE, et al. Cells and molecules which regulate B lymphopoiesis in bone marrow. Ann Rev Immunol 1989; 7: 111-43.

105. Rothenberg E, Lugo JP. Differentiation and cell division in the mammalian thymus. Dev Biol. 1985; 112: 1-8.

106. Weissman IL, Levy R. In vitro cortisone sensitivity of in vivo cortisone resistant thymocytes. Isr J Med Sci 1975; 11: 884-89.

107. Weissman IL, Baird S, Gardner RL, et al. Normal and neoplastic maturation of T-lineage lymphocytes. II. Cold Spring Harbor Symp. Quant. Biol. 1977; 41: 9-15.

108. Russell JH. Internal disintegration model of cytotoxic lymphocyte-induced damage. Immunol Rev 1983; 72: 97-117.

109. Ucker DS. Cytotoxic T lymphocytes and glucocorticoids activate an endogenous suicide process in target cells. Nature 1987; 327: 62-64.

110. Despont JP, Abel CA, Grey HM. Sialic acids and sialyl transferases in murine lymphoid cells: Indicators of T-cell maturation. Cell Immunol 1975; 17: 487-93.

111. Raedler A, Raedler E, Becker WM, et al. Subcapsular thymic lymphoblasts expose receptors for soybean lectin. Immunology 46: 1982; 231-38.

112. Rouse RV, Weissman IL. Microanatomy of the thymus: Its relationship to T-cell differentiation. Ciba Found Symp 1981; 84: 161-82.

113. Rouse RV, van Ewijk W, Jones PP, et al. Expression of MHC antigens by mouse thymic dendritic cells. J Immunol 1979; 122: 2508-12.

114. van Ewijk W, Rouse RV, Weissman IL. Distribution of H-2 microenvironments in the mouse thymus. J Histochem Cytochem 28: 1980; 1089-97.

115. Rouse RV, Parham P, Grumet FC, et al. Expression of HLA antigens by human thymic epithelial cells. Hum Immunol 1982; 5: 21-27.

116. Reichert RV, Gallatin WM, Butcher EC, et al. A homing receptor-bearing cortical thymocyte subset: Implications for thymus cell migration and the nature of cortisone-resistant thymocytes. Cell 1984; 38: 89-97.

117. Naparstek Y, Holoshitz J, Eisenstein S, et al. Effector T lymphocyte line cells migrate to the thymus and persist there. Nature 1982; 300: 262-65.

118. Fink PJ, Bevan MJ, Weissman IL. Thymic cytotoxic T lymphocytes are primed *in* vivo to minor histocompatibility antigens. J Exp Med 1984; 159: 436-47.

119. Michie SA, Kirkpatrick EA, Rouse RV. Rare peripheral T cells migrate to and persist in normal mouse thymus. J Exp Med 1988; 168: 1929-34.

120. Agus DB, Surh CD, Sprent J. Reentry of T cells to the adult thymus is restricted to activated T cells. J Exp Med 1991; 1039-46.

121. Rouse RV, Reichert RA, Gallatin WM, et al. Localization of lymphocyte subpopulations in peripheral lymphoid organs: Directed lymphocyte migration and segregation into specific microenvironments. Am J Anat 1984; 170: 391-99.

CHAPTER 6

DiGeorge's Syndrome
(Thymic Aplasia, Hypoplasia and Dysplasia)

Congenital thymic hypoplasia occurs as part of DiGeorge's syndrome, which is a congenital immunodeficiency disease caused by the maldevelopment of structures that are derived from the first through the sixth branchial pouches during embryonic development.[1-3] Structures derived from these branchial pouches include portions of the ear[4] and certain facial features (underdevelopment of the mandible, low-set ears, and ocular hypertelorism) (Fig. 1),[4] portions of the aortic arch and heart (resulting in truncus arteriosus, interrupted aortic arch, and tetralogy of Fallot),[5] the parathyroids[1] and thyroid,[3] and the thymus.[3] To be classified as the DiGeorge syndrome, the disorder must include both hypocalcemic tetany secondary to the parathyroid deficiency (with the lack of parathyroid hormone) and increased susceptibility to infections secondary to absence of cell-mediated immune responses (due to the lack of the thymus). The other features may or may not be present. Most cases appear to be familial involving autosomal recessive genes. Several chromosomal abnormalities have been reported in association with the DiGeorge anomaly, particularly monosomy 22q11 (Fig. 2).[6] Overall the percentage of chromosomal abnormalities, including monosomy 22q11, seen in association with the DiGeorge anomaly is approximately 15%.[6] A case of apparent autosomal dominant transmission of the DiGeorge anomaly has also been associated with monosomy 22q11.[7] The sexes are equally affected.

Between the 6th and 10th weeks of intrauterine life, the thymus, thyroid, parathyroids, and certain facial and vascular structures develop from elements of the first through sixth branchial pouches.[8] At about the twelfth week, the thymus begins to migrate to its final location in the thorax. An insult to the fetus during this critical time of development can lead to abnormalities in development of the structures derived from these embryonic tissues. Infants with the fetal alcohol syndrome may have facial abnormalities similar to those seen in the complete DiGeorge's syndrome, suggesting that ethanol may be one of the causative factors for this congenital abnormality.[9]

Patients with DiGeorge's syndrome usually present in early infancy with symptoms unrelated to immunodeficiency. Congenital heart defects, including truncus arteriosus, ventricular septal defect, interrupted aortic arch, and tetralogy of Fallot, are common presenting problems during the first two weeks of life.[5] Neural crest cells participate in the embryonic development of the aortopulmonary and conotruncal septa, the thymus and the parathyroid glands.[10] The recognition of a clinical syndrome with associated developmental anomalies of these tissues, the DiGeorge or "third and fourth nasopharyngeal pouch" syndrome, suggested a causal relation for an abnormality of neural-crest development.[5] In infants, a lateral chest x-ray or CT scan will determine the absence or dysplasia (thinness) of the thymus. Abnormal calcium homeostasis because of hypoparathyroidism is seen in all

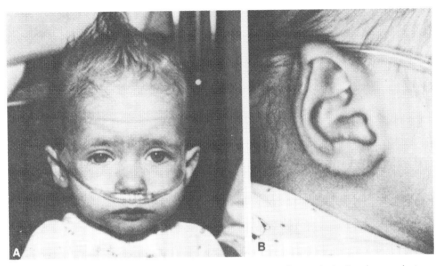

Fig. 1. Facial abnormalities of a child with DiGeorge's syndrome including hypertelorism, defective low set ears, hypoplastic mandible, and upward bowing of the upper lip (A). Close-up of the ear demonstrates notched pinna and deficient helix formation (B). [From Blaese RM, Hong R. Combined Immunodeficiency Diseases. In: Oski FA, ed. Principles of Pediatrics. 1st ed., Philadelphia: JB Lippincott, 1990:191.]

Fig. 2. Schematic representation of the short arm and proximal long arm of chromosome 22 that is lost in the DiGeorge syndrome probanes with unbalanced translocations of chromosome 22. Remaining long-arm material (q11→qter) translocates to an autosome. [From Fibison WJ, et al. 1990. Molecular studies of DiGeorge syndrome. Am J Hum Genetics 46: 888-895.]

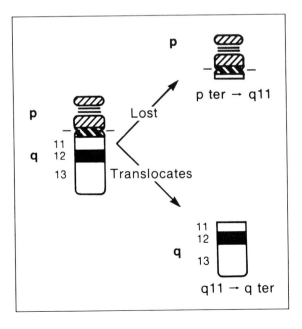

patients, and hypocalcemic tetany is the most common initial problem in patients presenting after the first month of life.[11] Facial abnormalities include microstomia, hypertelorism, upturned nose, posteriorly rotated small low-set ears with notched pinnae and an anti-Mongoloid slant of the eyes.[4,12] Runting, hypothyroidism, esophageal atresia, tracheoesophageal fistula and a bifid uvula have also been described in these patients.[13] If these patients survive this early period, they begin to experience an increased susceptibility to infections, including recurrent pneumonia, diarrhea, and candidiasis of the mouth, oropharynx, esophagus, and skin of the diaper area.[14]

DiGeorge's syndrome is extremely variable in the extent of its clinical manifestations and the degree of immunodeficiency. The immunologic defects in these patients are the direct consequence of the failure of thymus development and vary from severe deficiency at one extreme to normal immunity at the other. The total lymphocyte count may vary from severely depressed to normal T-cell levels but are usually more consistently depressed and may be less than 1% of normal.[13] Circulating lymphocytes in the affected patient usually only bear cell surface markers characteristic of prothymocytes, i.e., CD10, while the determinants characteristic of mature T cells, e.g., CD3, CD4, and CD8, are lacking. The morphology of the periarteriolar sheath of the spleen and the paracortical areas of the lymph nodes also reflects the T lymphopenia expected with thymic hypoplasia since both of these lymphoid deposits are considered to be the "thymic dependent areas".[14] Patients with severe thymic defects commonly will have no cutaneous delayed hypersensitivity reaction, skin-test anergy, and allow prolonged skin-allograft survival, as well as deficient in vitro T-cell proliferation to nonspecific antigens.[14] Other patients, however, may have normal T lymphocyte numbers and normal in vitro functional tests. Since B lymphocyte numbers and function are preserved, most patients[14] are able to make normal antibody responses after primary immunization. However, occasionally immunoglobulin levels can be low due to defective antibody synthesis. It is of great clinical importance that malignant tumors of the hematopoietic system, especially malignant lymphoma, occur 100 times more frequently in children with primary immunodeficiency than in those with healthy immune systems.[13]

Serial studies of immune function have shown that some patients with the partial form of DiGeorge syndrome clearly demonstrate a spontaneous improvement in immune function with time, while others have shown deterioration. Autopsy studies have shown that in two thirds of cases a small residue fragment of thymus with preserved architecture can be found, often in an ectopic location.[5] This variability in the degree of thymic deficiency appears to account for the variable pattern of clinical immune deficiency seen in this syndrome, and probably also accounts for those patients who seem to have only the nonimmunologic features of this syndrome.

The nonimmunologic features of this syndrome are often more life-threatening to newborns than is the immunodeficiency and initial treatment is directed at controlling the congenital heart disease and the metabolic abnormalities found in these infants.[5] Hypoparathyroidism and the associated hypocalcemia may require long-term replacement with vitamin D and calcium. The congenital heart disease is frequently severe, and often requires immediate surgical intervention.

Immunologic reconstitution of these patients has been attempted, using several different approaches including grafts of fetal thymus,[15,16] thymus tissue enclosed in a semipermeable chamber,[17] HLA-matched bone marrow transplantation,[18,19] and thymic humoral factors.[20] Success and failures have been experienced with each approach, but no generally accepted form of treatment has emerged, perhaps because of the great variability from patient to patient in the degree of thymic deficiency and the unpredictable course that many of these patients follow.

References

1. Lobdell DH. Congenital absence of the parathyroid glands. Arch Pathol Lab Med 1959; 67: 412-16.
2. DiGeorge AM. Discussions on a new concept of the cellular basis of immunity. J Pediatr 1965; 67: 907-08.
3. Lischner HW. DiGeorge syndrome(s). J Pediatr 1972; 81: 1042-44.
4. Conley ME, Beckwith JB, Mancer JFK, et al. The spectrum of the DiGeorge syndrome. J Pediatr 1979; 94: 883-90.
5. Lodewyk HS, Mierop V, Kutsche LM. Cardiovascular anomalies in DiGeorge syndrome and importance of neural crest as a possible pathogenic factor. Am J Cardiol 1986; 58: 133-38.
6. Greenberg F, Elder FF, Haffner P, et al. Cytogenic findings in a prospective series of patients with Digeorge anomaly. Am J Hum Genet 1988; 43: 605-11.
7. Greenberg F, Crowder WE, Paschall V, et al. Familial DiGeorge syndrome and associated partial monosomy of chromosome 22. Hum Genet 1984; 65: 317-19.
8. Lischner HW, Punnett HH, DiGeorge AM. Lymphocytes in congenital absence of the thymus. Nature. 1967; 214: 580-82.
9. Greenberg F. Hypoparathyroidism and the DiGeorge syndrome. N Engl J Med 1989; 320: 1146-52.
10. Kirby ML, Bockman DE. Neural crest and normal development: A new perspective. Anat Rec 1984; 209: 1-9.
11. Muller W, Peter HH, Wilken M. The DiGeorge syndrome. I. Clinical evaluation and course of partial and complete forms of the syndrome. Eur J Pediatr. 1988; 147: 496-503.
12. Stevens CA, Carey JC, Shigeoka AO. DiGeorge anomaly and velocardiofacial syndrome. Pediatrics 1990; 85: 526-32.
13. Rosen FS, Cooper MD, Wedgewood RJ. The primary immunodeficiencies (1). N Engl J Med 1984; 311: 235-41.
14. Rosen FS, Cooper MD, Wedgewood RL. The primary immunodeficiencies (2). N Engl J Med 1984; 311: 311-23.
15. August CS, Levey RH, Berkel AI, et al. Establishment of immunological competence in a child with congenital thymic aplasia by a graft of fetal thymus. Lancet 1970; 1: 1080-84.
16. Cleveland WW, Fogel BJ, Brown WT, et al. Fetal thymic transplant in a case of DiGeorge's syndrome. Lancet 1968; 2: 1211-16.
17. Steele RW, Limas C, Thurman GB, et al. Familial thymic aplasia: attempted reconstitution with fetal thymus in a millipore diffusion chamber. N Engl J Med 1972; 287: 787-92.

18. Goldsobel AB, Haas A, Stiehm ER. Bone marrow transplantation in DiGeorge syndrome. J Pediatr 1987; 111: 40-48.

19. Borzy MS, Ridgeway D, Noya FJ, et al. Successful bone marrow transplantation with split lymphoid chimerism in DiGeorge syndrome. J Clin Immunol 1989; 9: 386-93.

20. Ammann HJ, Hong R. Disorders of the T-cell system. In: Stiehm ER, ed. Immunologic Disorders in Infants and Children. 3rd ed. Philadelphia: WB Saunders, 1989: 257-313.

CHAPTER 7

THYMIC MICROENVIRONMENT, CYTOKINES AND HORMONES

HOW THE THYMIC MICROENVIRONMENT FUNCTIONS

The thymus is a rapidly proliferating primary lymphoid organ with the ability to maintain a defined microenvironment and appears to be essential for the production of mature T cells. Abnormalities of the thymus result in impaired T-cell immune responses. Thymic function is dependent upon interactions between developing thymocytes, outside factors (neural input, blood-borne factors), paracrine effects (intercellular interactions within the thymus), and feedback mechanisms (to the central nervous system and other organs). These interactions are complex and the concepts considered here are rapidly evolving areas in physiology.

The concept of neurotransmitters as products of neurons that interact with other neurons or cell types has been paralleled by the term "immunotransmitter" for immune system molecules that communicate with other cells.[1] It is now established that immunotransmitters also function in the central nervous system and that numerous peptides from the hypothalamic-pituitary axis (HPA) are immunoregulatory centrally and peripherally. Of particular importance is the demonstration of the synthesis and release of proopiomelanocortin (POMC) and growth hormone peptides from circulating lymphocytes[2,3] and the production of cytokines such as IL-1 (usually released by macrophages) by glial cells.[4] IL-1 is a potent activator of the HPA, especially affecting adrenocorticotrophic hormone (ACTH) and corticosterone.[5] While these interactions are of fundamental importance for the body's response to antigens, CNS/thymic communication research has been directed towards defining hypothalamic-pituitary influences on the thymus, neural pathways, chemoattraction, cytokine reactions, thymic hormones, relationships with other endocrine organs and with the CNS.

HYPOTHALAMIC AND PITUITARY INFLUENCES ON THE THYMUS

The hypothalamus is of primary importance in the control of the endocrine and autonomic nervous systems. It is also structurally and functionally related to the higher regions of the nervous system and may be the main center through which behavioral events, e.g., those causing stress, affect the neuroendocrine-immune system. In addition, the suprachiasmatic nucleus appears to be the biological clock or endogenous pacemaker in animals, and many factors and hormones (including those of the immune response) have circadian rhythms of release. Thus the type of immune response and its efficiency is influenced by and, in turn affects, hypothalamic events.[6]

Evidence for direct interactions between the hypothalamus/pituitary axis and the thymus was presented when the prosencephalon and primordium of the chick embryo's hypophysis were removed at 33-38 hours of incubation. This resulted in involution of the thymus and fewer peripheral lymphocytes.[7] Thymic involution occurring after hypophysectomy or lesions of the rodent preoptic anterior hypothalamic area[8] influenced immune function. In contrast, anterior pituitary growth hormone given to hypophysectomized animals produced a great increase in thymic weight.[9]

Experimental thymectomy,[10] or the athymic state as in the hypopituitary dwarf mouse[11] is accompanied by degranulation of the anterior pituitary cells producing growth hormone and prolactin.[12] When antigrowth hormone antibodies are given to intact young mice, a wasting disease is produced that is similar to that seen after thymectomy.[13] These effects could be reversed by growth hormone or thyroxine treatment.[14] At an early age, hypopituitary dwarf mice lack thymulin biological activity.[15] Prolactin, as well as growth and thyroid hormones, all increase the secretion of thymic hormones[16] in vivo and in vitro. Abnormalities of pituitary hormones observed in patients with hypo- and hyperthyroidism, pituitary dwarfism and acromegaly[17,18] are similar to those found with the experimental manipulations of thymulin levels outlined above.

ACTH from the pituitary acts primarily on the adrenal cortex to cause the release of adrenocortical steroids, mainly cortisol, which in high doses causes thymocyte death by apoptosis. Recently, however, it has been shown that in vivo and in vitro ACTH also releases thymulin which may protect the immune system in acute stress.

THYMIC CHEMOATTRACTANTS

The thymus is known to attract prothymocytes, circulating stem cells or pre-T cells. One such chemotaxic peptide, previously called thymotaxin, has been extensively studied (reviewed in 19). Substances purified from embryonic mouse thymus epithelium possessed both a chemotaxic (m.w. 4 kDa) and a chemokinetic function (<5 kDa). The chemotaxic factor (thymotaxin) with activity on hemopoietic precursors from the bone marrow was finally demonstrated to have a m.w. of 11 kDa. This molecule has recently been identified as β2 microglobulin (the light chain of MHC class I and CD1 molecules).[20] Cells responding to this molecule are resting cells (probably committed to the T lineage), high in their expression of Thy-1, low in T- and B-cell differentiation markers and do not proliferate under the influence of IL-1 or IL-3 stimulation. After three days in culture, thymotaxin treatment resulted in significant expression of CD8 and CD4 on pre-T cells.[19]

THYMIC CYTOKINES

Once prothymocytes are within the thymus cortex, they are exposed to the influences of a wide variety of secreted factors. Cytokines from thymic epithelial cells include IL-1, IL-4 and colony stimulating factor for macrophages (CSF-M); from macrophages IL-1, IL-6, IL-7, TNF-α and CSF-M; and from endothelial cells IL-1, IL-6 and CSF-M.[21] Most other known cytokines could be involved in a minor way, since the thymus can contain a wide variety of different cell types at different times. When specialized situations occur, they reflect a property of the thymus, e.g., when eosinophils are found to develop in the thymus, IL-5 is probably involved. In addition, thymocytes themselves secrete IL-1, IL-2, IL-4, IL-6, IL-7, IFN-γ and lymphotoxin or TNF-β during the different stages of T-cell ontogeny.[22] When activated, mature T cells can also secrete TNF-α.[21]

Some principles have emerged from the bewildering array of possible interactions. In general, the interactions within the thymus appear to be very specific and limited to short-range communications where cells may actually be touching.[23] This has been elegantly shown by the electron microscopy of Farr et al[24] and von Gaudecker et al.[25] Thus immense immune response variability can be evoked depending on the repertoire of receptor expression on the responding cells. Down- or up-regulation of receptor expression may also provide an exquisite method of controlling cellular interactions whose dynamics can be further modulated by other events such as hormonal actions.

Within the thymus of the 14-day fetal mouse, the differentiation, but not proliferation, of early thymocytes and in adults of CD4⁻/CD8⁻ double negative cells is under the control of IL-7.[26] IL-4 is also important in the growth and differentiation of murine thymocytes up to 16 days of gestation[27] but a costimulus is required for a response.[28] While double negative thymocytes also proliferate in vitro under the influence of IL-1,[29] in vivo this immune response also always requires another stimulator such as a mitogen. The cytokine IL-2 (produced in vivo by other double negative thymocytes, macrophages and mature T cells) acts on peripheral T-cell IL-2 receptors to amplify clonal expansion during the immune response. Thymocytes also have been shown to specifically bear receptors for IL-2 during the early stages of thymocyte ontogeny of double negative (CD4⁻/CD8⁻) cells. These IL-2 receptor bearing cells show a greater propensity to enter mitosis and differentiate to mature T cells[30, 31] than do IL-2 receptor negative double negative thymocytes. The use of anti-IL-2 antibodies has been shown to block proliferation and expression of the αβ T-cell receptor of differentiating thymocytes.[32] Despite this, a functional role for the IL-2 receptor has been questioned in certain in vitro experiments.[33] IL-6 is another cytokine with proliferative and differentiation properties especially in synergistic combination with IL-2 and IL-4. For example, IL-6 may act to prepare cells to express IL-2 receptor on thymocytes.[34] Both IL-2 and IL-4 may also be involved in repertoire selection and expression of differentiation antigens. IL-2 induces the development of CD3⁺/αβ T-cell receptor positive cells, and IL-4 enhances the expression of Thy-1 and CD45 (high-molecular weight) antigen on mature postthymic T cells.[34]

Although intrathymic events may result from locally produced cytokines, immune challenge elsewhere in the body may alter thymic function by releasing circulating levels of cytokines that have systemic effects. For example, systemic administration of IL-1 is known to release ACTH (amongst other things).[5] ACTH is a potent releaser of the thymic hormone thymulin,[21] and thymulin has been demonstrated to induce T-cell differentiation markers on prethymic cells and to influence the production of CD8[+] T cells. This is only one of the many possible neuroimmunoendocrine interactions thought to act on lymphopoiectic events.

THYMIC HORMONES

The thymus produces a number of peptides which appear to act within the thymus in a paracrine fashion and in the systemic circulation as feedback signals to the central nervous system.[35] There are four well-defined and apparently unrelated thymic peptides will be considered here: thymosin α1, thymopoietin, thymulin, and thymic hormonal factor. Recent reviews on their biology and methods of assay detail their structure and general characteristics.[36,37] The structure of thymic hormonal factor has been published.[38]

Thymosins

Thymosin α1 was isolated and purified by Low et al[39] from a complex mixture of 40-50 polypeptides called thymosin faction 5 (TF5), and shown to be secreted by single or grouped subcapsular epithelial cells, and cells around Hassel's corpuscles.[40] The presence of thymosin α1 in the arcuate nucleus and median eminence of the central nervous system[41] has led to it being ascribed a role in neuroimmunomodulation.[1] It has been suggested that it is a proteolytic fragment of a larger native polypeptide, prothymosin α1 that has been isolated from the thymus (highest concentrations), spleen, lung, kidney and brain.[42] Thymosin α1 has a wide range of immunomodulatory effects ascribed to it, including inducing the differentiation of murine cortical thymocytes, modulating terminal deoxynucleotidyl-transferase (TdT) expression, stimulating lymphocyte mitogen responses and enhancing production of interferon and macrophage migration inhibitory factor.[43]

In most clinical studies using TF5 (mixture of polypeptides), there are generally significant improvements in T-cell numbers and functions, decreased infections, increased weight gain, and overall clinical improvement. It is nevertheless important to determine the action of individual peptides. For example, the intraperitoneal injection of TF5, but not thymosin α1, causes a dose-dependent increase in serum corticosterone in rodents.[44]

Thymosin α1 plasma concentrations are lowered in immunodeficiency conditions and in adults with malignancy[45,46] but raised in pediatric acquired immunodeficiency syndrome (AIDS) and AIDS-related complex.[47-49] These latter observations may be erroneous, however, since there is some sequence homology between thymosin α1 and proteins of different isolates of human immunodeficiency virus (HIV).[50]

Recently a thymic peptide, MB-35, was also purified, chemically synthesized and sequenced from TF5.[51] It has sequence homology with residues 86-120 of the nuclear histone H2A previously isolated from the thymus. It is more potent than TF5 in the stimulation of prolactin and growth hormone release from anterior pituitary cells in vitro.

The amino-acid sequence of thymosin B₄ (which is not an exclusive thymic hormone) has been established.[52] It is probably active in the early stages of thymocyte differentiation as it induces the enzyme terminal deoxynucleotidyl transferase in murine thymocytes in vitro and in vivo.

This thymic hormone also stimulates the hypothalamic secretion of luteinizing hormone releasing factor which in turn causes the pituitary to release luteinizing hormone.[53]

Thymopoietin

Thymopoietin, like its synthetic pentapeptide thymopentin, induces early T-cell differentiation and regulates the function of T cells[54, 55] although it was primarily recognized for its detrimental effects on neuromuscular transmission. It is probably produced by epithelial cells of the thymus.[56] Ubiquitin found in most body tissues, and splenin from lymph nodes and spleen, are related peptides with distinctly different biological roles. Splenin, for example, does not affect neuromuscular transmission, although it only differs from thymopoietin by one amino acid substitution. Both the synthetic pentapeptide thymopentin and native thymopoietin bind with high affinity to the acetylcholine receptor. It has been postulated that autoimmune thymitis in myasthenia gravis results in the hypersecretion of thymopoietin and consequent impairment of acetylcholine-mediated transmission at the neuromuscular junction.[57] The demonstration of acetylcholine receptors in the human thymus supports the view that the origins of this disease are in the thymus.[58] Recently Kendall and Ritter reported identifying a 153 kDa molecular weight protein in thymomas of myasthenia gravis patients which shares antigenic determinants with the muscle acetylcholine receptor.[59] Perhaps this antigen will be shown to trigger the autoimmune myasthenia gravis.

Thymopoietin has been used to modify autoimmunity in animal models. Lau et al[60] found that when thymopoietin was injected there was a faster loss of autoantibodies to injected cross-reacting rat erythrocytes than in control mice. There was also a delay in the appearance of autoantibodies when spleen cells from mice immunized with rat erythrocytes were transferred to syngeneic recipients undergoing similar immunization schedules.

Thymulin

Thymulin was isolated and characterized as "facteur thymique serique" from porcine serum.[61] It is a well-conserved nonapeptide without species specificity that is produced by epithelial cells of the subcapsular cortex and medulla in the thymus, circulates in the blood bound to unidentified carriers and requires zinc for its biological activity. Thymulin binds to high affinity membrane receptors and induces T-cell markers on bone marrow cells and CD3[+] and Lyt2[+] cells in the mouse.[62,63] Thymulin also affects mature T cells, particularly of the CD8[+] subset in a concentration dependent manner. CD3[+], CD4[+] or CD8[+] antigens are modulated when thymulin is given to humans with immune deficiencies.[64]

The precise characterization of the action of thymulian has been hampered by the lack of a reliable quantitative assay. By the existing bioassay, blood thymulin activity is reduced in immunodeficiencies[65,46,48] and in aging healthy adults. In children with AIDS or AIDS-related complex abnormally low plasma levels of thymulin precedes the development of peripheral blood T-cell abnormalities.[48] Hypothyroidism and diabetes are also associated with low levels of serum thymulin activity and treatment with the appropriate dose of thyroid hormone or insulin, respectively, restored thymulin levels to normal. As expected, hyperthyroid patients have higher than normal levels of thymulin.[66] These observations and experimental manipulations suggest that both thyroid hormones and insulin are required for the continued output of thymulin and that the decreases levels observed with aging can be reversed. Use of a quantitative radioimmunoassay shows that thymulin levels are highest in neonates, reduced in youngsters before 20 years of age and remain low throughout adulthood.[67] Preliminary work with the autoimmune condition, alopecia areata, shows that these patients also have significantly lowered plasma thymulin levels.[21]

Research currently is directed at understanding the relationship between blood thymulin levels and thymocyte function. Preliminary results indicate that both low and high thymulin levels have been associated with a low percentage of CD8+ cells in the thymus and to a lesser extent in the periphery.[68] Thymulin appears to be a potent inhibitor of suppressor T cells in the periphery[69] by unknown mechanisms.

Thymulin release can also fluctuate. Thymulin levels followed in four surgical patients were consistently reduced during surgery but rose during the recovery period to levels greater than those measured at the induction of anaesthesia in a pattern similar to that of cortisol and ACTH.[70] When thymulin release by incubates of thymic tissue, stimulated by physiological levels of ACTH in adrenalectomized young rats (which also removed endogenous corticosterone with stress levels of ACTH) were measured, there was a significant hypersecretion of thymulin which could be mimicked by potassium administration and was calcium dependent.[71] Some peptides coreleased with ACTH have also been shown to elevate thymulin release from cultured cells.[72] Thus ACTH, the major pituitary factor released during stress, has an important functional role in increasing the secretion of thymulin, which in turn influences the immune status.

Thymic Humoral Factor

Thymic humoral factor was initially characterized by Trainin and Small[73] and used as a crude extract to restore the immune competence of lymphoid cells from neonatally thymectomized mice. Injection of the thymic humoral factor protected the mice from wasting disease and allowed them to reject tumors and allogeneic skin grafts.[74] Thymic humoral factor is essential for induction of clonal expansion, differentiation and maturation of T-cell subsets. It also augments most T-cell functions and has been used clinically to normalize CD4/CD8 ratios in severe viral infections, after intensive chemotherapy for malignant disease, and with autoimmune disease.[75]

HORMONES FROM OTHER ENDOCRINE GLANDS

There is evidence that all the major hormones released from endocrine organs can influence thymic events and/or structure. Adrenal and gonadal hormones have the most potent effects, generally causing thymocyte apoptosis and reduced thymic weight. The increased thymus weight with both gonadectomy and adrenalectomy is quite striking in aging animals.[59] While thymocytes bear receptors for glucocorticoids, prothymocytes are the most susceptible to glucocorticoid action and medullary thymocytes are the most resistant. The sex hormones probably act through the microenvironment since specific high affinity estrogen receptors, for example, are found on epithelial cells but not on thymocytes. Hypertrophy of epithelial cells is seen after thyroxine treatment.[76] Functionally this results in more thymulin-secreting cells in the gland and increased serum thymulin levels, although no receptors have yet been observed for the metabolite of thyroxine, T_3.[77]

It is apparent that the thymus has a dynamic microenvironment which can vary with physiological conditions such as aging, and can respond rapidly to a variety of events such as stress, viral infection and chemical toxicity. The constantly changing cellular dynamics of the thymus need to be carefully appraised to understand the impact of a fully functional thymus on immune function throughout life.

REFERENCES

1. Hall NR, McGillis JP, Spangelo BL, et al. Evidence that thymosins and other biological response modifiers can function as neuroactive immunotransmitters. J Immunol 1985;135: 806-11.

2. Blalock JE, Harbour-McMenamin D, Smith EM. Peptide hormones shared by the neuroendocrine and immunologic systems. J Immunol 1985; 135: 858-61.

3. Weigent D, Blalock JE. Growth hormone and the immune system. Prog Neuro Endocr Immun 1990;3: 231-41.

4. Fontana A, Kristensen F, Dubs R, et al. Production of prostaglandin E and an interleukin-1-like factor by cultured astrocytes and C6 glioma cells. J Immunol 1982;129: 2413-19.

5. Dunn AJ. Interleukin-1 as a stimulator of hormone secretion. Progress in Neuro Endocrine Immunol 1990;3: 26-34.

6. Besedovsky H, Sorkin E, Felix D, et al. Hypothalamic changes during the immune response. Eur J Immunol 1977; 7: 323-25.

7. Jankovic BD, Isakovic K, and Knezevic Z. Ontogeny of the immuno-neuro-endocrine relationship. Changes in lymphoid tissue of chick embryos surgically decapitated at 33-38 hours of incubation. Developmental and Comparative Immunology 1979; 2: 479-94.

8. Knutson F, Lundin PM. The effect of hypophysectomy, adrenalectomy and cortisone on the incorporation of tritiated thymidine in rat organs, with special reference to the lymphoid organs. Acta Endocrinologica 1966; 53: 519-26.

9. Shrewsbury MM, Reinhardt WO. Effect of pituitary growth on lymphatic tissues, thoracic duct lymph flow, lymph protein and lymphocyte output in the rat. Endocrinology 1959; 65: 858-60.

10. Pierpaoli W, Bianchi E, Sorkin E. Hormones and the immunological capacity. V. Modification of growth hormone producing cells in the adenohypophysis of neonatally thymectomized germ-free mice: an electron microscopic study. Clin Exp Immun 1971; 9: 889-901.

11. Fabris N, Pierpaoli W, Sorkin E. Hormones and immunological capacity. III. The immunodeficiency disease of the hypopituitary Snell-Bagg mouse. Clin Exp Immun 1971; 9: 209-25.

12. Bianchi E, Pierpaoli W, Sorkin E. Cytological changes in the mouse anterior pituitary after neonatal thymectomy: a light and electron microscopical study. J Endocrinol 1971; 51: 1-6.

13. Pierpaoli W, Sorkin E. Hormones and immunological capacity. I. Effect of heterologous antigrowth hormone (ASTH) antiserum on thymus and periph-

eral lymphatic tissue in mice. Induction of wasting syndrome. J Immunol 1968; 101: 1036-43.

14. Pierpaoli W, Barboni C, Fabris N, et al. Hormones and the immunologic capacity. II. Reconstitution of antibody production in hormonally deficient mice by somatotropic hormone, thyrotrophic hormone and thyroxine. Immunology 1969; 16: 217-30.

15. Pelletier M, Montplaisir S, Dardenne M, et al. Thymic hormone activity and spontaneous autoimmunity in dwarf mice and their littermates. Immunolology 1976; 30: 783-88.

16. Dardenne M, Savino W. Neuroendocrine control of the thymic epithelium: modulation of thymic endocrine function, cytokine expression and cell proliferation by hormones and peptides. Prog Neuro Endocrin Immun 1990; 3: 18-25.

17. Fabris N, Mocchfgiani E, Pacini F, et al. Thyroid function modulates thymic endocrine activity. J Clin Endocrin Metab 1986; 62: 474-78.

18. Timsit J, Safieh B, Gagnerault MC, et al. Augmentation des taux circulantes de thymuline au cours de l'hyperprolactinemie et de l'acromegalie. Compte Rendu de l'Academie des Sciences (Paris) 1990; 31(III): 7-13.

19. Imhof BA, Deugnier MA, Bauvois B, et al. Properties of the pre-T cells and their chemotactic migration to the thymus. Thymus Update 1989; 2: 3-19.

20. Dargemont C, Dunon D, Deugnier M, et al. Thymotaxin, a chemotactic protein is identical to β2-microglobulin. Science 1989; 246: 803-06.

21. Kendall MD. Functional anatomy of the thymic microenvironment. J Anat 1991; 177: 1-29.

22. Montgomery RA, Dallman MJ. Analysis of cytokine gene expression during fetal thymic ontogeny using the polymerase chain reaction. J Immunol 1991; 147: 554-60.

23. Poo WJ, Conrad L, Janeway CA. Receptor directed focusing of lymphokine release by T helper cells. Nature 1988; 332: 378-80.

24. Farr AG, Anderson SK, Marrack P, et al. Expression of antigen-specific major histocompatibility complex-restricted receptors by cortical and medullary thymocytes in situ. Cell 1985; 43: 543-50.

25. Gaudecker B von, Larche M, Schuurman HJ, et al. Analysis of the fine distribution of thymic epithelial microenvironment molecules by immunoelectron microscopy. Thymus 1989; 13: 187-94.

26. Henney CS. Interleukin-7: Effects on early events in lymphopoiesis. Immunology Today 1989; 10: 170-73.

27. Sideras P, Funa K, Zalcberg-Quintana I, et al. Analysis by in situ hybridization of cells expressing mRNA for interleukin-4 in the developing thymus and in peripheral lymphocytes from mice. Proc Natl Acad Sci USA 1988; 85: 218-21.

28. Zlotnik A, Ransom J, Frank G, et al. Interleukin-4 is a growth factor for activated thymocytes: possible role in T-cell ontogeny. Proc Natl Acad Sci USA 1987; 84: 3856-60.

29. Chaudhari G, Clark IA, Ceredig R. Proliferation in vivo of Lyt2-, L3T4- thymocytes shows responsiveness to interleukin-1. Clin Exp Immunol 1988; 73: 51-56.

30. Gearing AJH, Wadhwa M, Perris AD. in vivo administration of interleukin-2 stimulates mitosis in thymus and bone marrow. Eur J Immunol 1986; 16: 1171-74.

31. Crispe IN. Thymocyte precursor-product relationships: close to a consensus. Thymus Update 1990; 3: 3-13.

32. Jenkinson EJ, Kingston R, Owen JJT. Importance of IL-2 receptors in in vitro thymic generation of cells expressing T receptors. Nature 1987; 329: 160-62.

33. Plum J, deSmedt M. Differentiation of thymocytes in fetal organ culture: lack of evidence for the functional role of interleukin receptor expressed by prothymocytes. Eur J Immunol 1988; 18: 795-99.

34. Hodgkin PD, Bond MW, O'Garra A, et al. Identification of IL-6 as a T-cell derived factor that enhances the proliferative response of thymocytes to IL-4 and phorbol myristate acetate. J Immunol 1988; 141: 151-57.

35. Trainin N. Thymic hormones and the immune response. Physiol Rev 1974; 54: 272-315.

36. Dardenne M, Bach JF. Functional biology of thymic hormones. Thymus Update 1988; 1: 101-16.

37. Safieh B, Kendall MD. Methods for assaying thymic hormones. Thymus Update 1988; 1: 117-33.

38. Burstein Y, Buchner V, Pecht M, et al. Thymic humoral factor γ 2: purification and amino acid sequence of an immunoregulatory peptide from calf thymus. Biochemistry 1988; 27: 4066-71.

39. Low TLK, Thurman GB, McAdoo M, et al. The chemistry and biology of thymosin. I. Isolation, characterization and biological activities of thymosin α1 and polypeptide α1 from calf thymus. J Biol Chem 1979; 254: 981-86.

40. Dalakas MC, Engel WK, McClure JE, et al. Immunocytochemical localization of thymosin α1 in thymic epithelial cells of normal and myasthenia gravis patients and in thymic cultures. J Neurol Sci 1981; 50: 239-47.

41. Palaszynski EW, Moody TW, O'Donohue TL, et al. Thymosin α1-like peptides: localization and biochemical characterization in the rat brain and pituitary gland. Peptides 1983; 4: 463-67.

42. Haritos AA, Tsolas O, Horecker BL. Distribution of prothymosin a in rat tissues. Proc Natl Acad Sci USA. 1984; 81: 1391-95.

43. Low TLK, Goldstein AL. Thymosins: isolation, structural studies, and biological activities. In: Silber R, Lobuc J, Gordon AS, eds. The Year in Hematology. New York: Plenum Press, 1984: 21-35.

44. McGillis JP, Hall NR, Vahouny GV, et al. Thymosin factor 5 causes increased serum corticosterone in rodents in vivo. J Immunol 1985; 134: 3952-55.

45. Wara DW, Martin NL, Wara WM. Thymosin α1 levels in children with primary cellular immunodeficiency and in adults with malignancy. In: Serrou B, ed. Current Concepts in Human Immunology and Cancer Immunomodulation. New York: Biomedical Press, 1982: 354-59.

46. Iwata T, Incefy CS, Good RA, et al. Circulating thymic hormone activity in patients with primary and secondary immunodeficiency disease. Am J Med 1983; 71: 385-94.

47. Hersch EM, Reuben JM, Rios A, et al. Elevated serum thymosin α1 levels associated with evidence of immune dysregulation in male homosexuals with a history of infectious diseases or Kaposi's sarcoma. N Engl J Med 1983; 308: 45-46.

48. Rubinstein R, Novick BE, Sicklick MJ, et al. Circulating thymulin and thymosin α1 activity in pediatric acquired immune deficiency syndrome: in vivo

and in vitro studies. J Peds 1986; 109: 422-27.

49. Naylor PH, Naylor CW, Badamchian M, et al. Human immunodeficiency virus contains an epitope immunoreactive with thymosin α1 and the 30 amino acid synthetic p17 group-specific antigen peptide HGP-30. Proc Natl Acad Sci USA 1987; 84: 2951-55.

50. Schuurman HJ, van Baarlem J, Krone WJA, et al. The thymus in the acquired immune deficiency syndrome. Thymus Update 1988; 1: 171-89.

51. Badamchian M, Wang SS, Spangelo BL, et al. Chemical and biological characterization of MB-35: a thymic derived peptide that stimulates the release of growth hormone and prolactin from rat anterior pituitary cells. Progress in NeuroEndocrinImmunology 1990; 3: 258-65.

52. Low TLK, Hu SK, Goldstein AL. Complete amino acid sequence of bovine thymosin *B*4: a thymic hormone that induces terminal deoxynucleotidyl transferase activity in thymocyte populations. Proc Natl Acad Sci USA 1981; 78: 1162-66.

53. Rebar RW, Miyake A, Low TLK, et al. Thymosin stimulates secretion of luteinizing hormone-releasing factor. Science 1981; 214: 669-71.

54. Goldstein G, Scheid MP, Boyse EA, et al. A synthetic pentapeptide with biological activity characteristic of the thymic hormone thymopoietin. Science 1979; 204: 1309-10.

55. Ranges GE, Goldstein G, Boyse EA, et al. T-cell development in normal and thymopoietin treated nude mice. J Exp Med 1982; 156: 1057-64.

56. Viamontes GI, Audhya T, Goldstein G. Immunohistochemical localization of thymopoietin with an antiserum to synthetic cys-thymopoietin$_{28-39}$. Cell Immunol 1986; 100: 305-13.

57. Venkatasubramanian K, Audhya T, Goldstein G. Binding of thymopoietin to the acetylcholine receptor. Proc Natl Acad Sci USA 1986; 83: 3171-74.

58. Raimond F, Morel E, Bach JF. Evidence for the presence of immunoreactive acetylcholine receptors on human thymus cells. J Neuroimmunol 1984; 6: 31-40.

59. Kendall MD, Ritter MA. The role of the thymus in tolerance induction. Thymus Update 1990; 3: 21-45.

60. Lau CY, Freestone JA, Goldstein G. Effect of thymopoietin pentapeptide (TP5) on autoimmunity. 1. TP5 suppression of induced erythrocyte autoantibodies in C3H mice. J Immunol 1980; 125: 1634-38.

61. Bach JF, Dardenne M, Pleau JM, et al. Biochemical characterization of a serum thymic factor. Nature 1976; 266: 55-56.

62. Bach JF, Dardenne M, Goldstein AL, et al. Appearance of T-cell markers in bone marrow rosette-forming cells after incubation with thymosin, a thymic hormone. Proc Natl Acad Sci USA 1971; 68: 2734-38.

63. Dardenne M, Charriere J, Bach JF. Alterations in thymocyte surface markers after in vivo treatment by serum thymic factor. Cellular Immunology (New York) 1978; 39: 47-54.

64. Bordigioni P, Faure G, Bene MC, et al. Improvement of cellular immunity and IgA production in immunodeficient children after treatment with synthetic serum thymic factor (FTS) Lancet 1982; II: 293-97.

65. Incefy GS, Dardenne M, Pahwa S, et al. Thymic activity in severe combined immunodeficiency diseases. Proc Natl Acad Sci USA 1977; 74: 1250-53.

66. Fabris N, Mocchegiani E. Endocrine control of thymic serum factor production in young adult and old mice. Cell Immunol 1985; 91: 325-35.

67. Safieh B, Kendall MD, Norman JC, et al. A new radioimmunoassay for the thymic peptide thymulin, and its application for measuring thymulin in blood samples. J Immunol Meth 1990; 127: 255-62.

68. Kendall MD, Safieh B, Sereen A, et al. Thymulin secreting cells in man: distribution, LM, histochemistry and plasma thymulin levels. In: Ritter MA, ed. Lymphatic Tissues and In Vivo Immune Responses. New York: Marcel Dekker, 1991: 234-54.

69. Bach JF, Bach MA, Charriere J, et al. The effect of the serum thymic factor (FTS) on suppressor T cells. In: Hadden J, Cherdid L, Mullen P, Spreafico F, eds. Advances in Immunopharmacology. Oxford: Pergamon Press, 1986: 77-81.

70. Chambers DJ, Karimzandi N, Braimbridge MV, et al. Hormone and electrolyte responses during and after open heart surgery. Thorac Cardiovasc Surg 1984; 32: 358-64.

71. Buckingham JC, Safieh B, Singh S, et al. Interactions of corticotropin and glucocorticoids in the control of thymulin release in the rat. Brit J Pharmacol 1991; 102: 15P.

72. Savino W, Gagnerault MC, Bach JF, et al. Neuroendocrine control of thymic hormonal production. II. Stimulatory effects of endogenous opioids on thymulin production by cultured human and murine thymic epithelial cells. Life Sciences 1990; 46: 1687-97.

73. Trainin N, Small M. Studies on some physiochemical properties of a thymus humoral factor conferring immunocompetence on lymphoid cells. J Exp Med 1970; 132: 885-89.

74. Trainin N, Rotter V, Yakir Y, et al. Biochemical and biological properties of THF in animals and human models. Ann NY Acad Sci1979; 332: 9-22.

75. Trainin N. Therapeutic properties of THF—thymic hormone—in autoimmune processes. Israel J Med Sci 1988; 24: 739-40.

76. Scheiff JM, Cordier AC, Haumont S. Epithelial cell proliferation in thymic hyperplasia induced by triiodothyronine. Clin Exp Immunol 1977; 27: 516-21.

77. Savino W, Wolf B, Aratan-Spire S, et al. Thymic hormone-containing cells. IV. Fluctuations in the thyroid hormone levels in vivo can modulate the secretion by human and murine epithelial cells. Clin Exp Immunol 1984; 55: 629-35.

CHAPTER 8

ONTOGENY OF THE T LYMPHOCYTE

S ince the early 1960s, when groups led by Jacques Miller, Robert Good and Byron Waksman demonstrated the critical influence of the thymus on the functioning of the immune system,[1] understanding of the function of the thymus in T lymphocyte development has increased steadily. Recently, studies have outlined certain differentiation pathways of T lymphocytes and in this section we will review the current thoughts on the intrathymic development of T cells.

THE EARLY PHASE OF DEVELOPMENT: DOUBLE NEGATIVE CELLS

T lymphocyte development within the thymus involves a complex pathway of thymocyte division and differentiation that is characterized by the acquisition and loss of specific cell surface antigens. Precursors of $\alpha\beta$ T cells colonize the murine thymus at about day 11 of fetal life[2,3] and continue to migrate into this organ throughout adult life.[3] T lymphocyte precursors originate in the bone marrow where they can be identified by the expression of Thy-1[lo] and Pgp-1+ (CD44+) (Fig. 1) but do not express the T-cell receptor (TCR). Upon emigration to the thymus, bone-marrow-derived prothymocytes are believed to undergo expansion and differentiation to a thymocyte population that does not express the cell surface differentiation molecule CD4 (L3T4) or CD8 (Lyt2) (double negative).[4,5]

Several years ago, Fowlkes et al[5] showed that the earliest intrathymic T-cell precursors are contained within a small fraction of thymocytes (2-3%) that express neither of the T-cell accessory molecules CD8 and CD4; that is, they are CD8⁻CD4⁻, double negative or DN. Intensive analysis has shown that DN thymocytes are heterogenous and several subsets have been characterized phenotypically and functionally.[6-15]

Initial studies have identified two classes of DN thymocytes distinguishable by their expression of heat-stable antigen.[16,17] From these studies, it was deduced that the bone marrow precursors express high levels of the heat-stable antigen (HSA+++) (immature thymocyte marker) soon after reaching the thymus and more than 90% of the population of DN thymocytes in young adult mice are HSA+++.[14] The minor fraction of DN cells that is HSA⁻ is composed of $\alpha\beta$ TCR+ thymocytes (predominately Vβ8+),[10,18] $\gamma\delta$ TCR+ thymocytes[8,11,12] and a few TCR⁻ Pgp-1+ cells which are the earliest

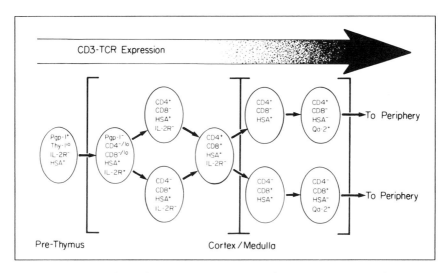

Fig. 1. A summary of the phenotype stages of T lymphocyte maturation in the thymus. Expression and localization of thymocyte subpopulations defined by the cell surface markers CD4, CD8, HSA, IL-2R, Qa-2 and Pgp-1 are shown. CD3-TCR expression is depicted by the arrow at top with increasing shading from left to right representing increasing CD3-TCR gene expression.

intrathymic precursor population.[7] The double-negative, HSA⁺ thymocytes give rise to immature single-positive thymocytes that express either the CD4 or CD8 molecule but not both.[19-22] After further expansion, these HSA⁺ single positive populations differentiate to CD4⁺CD8⁺HSA⁺ thymocytes.[23] (to be discussed in subsequent sections)

Both TCR⁺ subsets are functionally mature. γδ TCR⁺ DN cells are present in the thymus from early ontogeny (day 14-15)[11], whereas αβ TCR⁺ DN thymocytes are first detectable at about the third week of life and accumulate with age.[3] When transferred intrathymically, αβTCR⁺, HSA⁺ IL-2 receptor positive DN thymocytes can give rise to small but detectable numbers of these Vβ8⁺ DN thymocytes. A considerable body of evidence indicates that these DN cells may use an alternative, poorly defined, differentiation pathway[3,10] that does not follow the standard intrathymic selection rules.[18] Interestingly, some of the Vβ8⁺ DN cells also express natural killer (NK) cell markers.[24,25]

HSA⁺⁺⁺ DN thymocytes contain three subpopulations defined by the expression of Pgp-1 (a very early prothymocyte marker)[26,27] and IL-2 receptor (IL-2R). First, HSA⁺⁺⁺ Pgp-1⁺, IL-2R⁻ cells can readily home to the thymus when injected intravenously and take approximately two weeks to develop into mature, single positive thymocytes (CD8⁺ or CD4⁺).[7] α TCR genes are not rearranged in this population. A second very minor population of thymocytes begin to express the IL-2R (55 kDa subunit) while Pgp-1 expression is downregulated, but still present, so that both markers are expressed at any given time.[7] The third and dominant HSA⁺⁺⁺ DN subpopulation consists of thymocytes expressing IL-2R, but not Pgp-1, that can repopulate the thymus when injected intrathymically[15] or intravenously.[7] mRNA analysis has revealed that β,[28] but not α,[28,29] TCR chain genes are rearranged and transcribed in these cells.

AN EARLY INTERMEDIATE STAGE: CD8^{lo}CD4^{lo}TCR^{lo}

The most critical intracellular event in the maturation of a thymocyte is the expression of the TCR heterodimer on the cell surface. This expression can first be detected on thymocytes that originate from the HSA^{+++} IL-2R$^+$ DN cells (Fig. 1).[29] DN thymocytes express IL-2R[30-32] transiently[15] and its down-regulation is paralleled by the most dramatic changes in developing T cells. The TCR α chain mRNA appears in the cytoplasm[29] and the CD3-TCR complex is assembled and expressed on the cell surface at low levels.[29] CD8 and CD4 molecules are also expressed at low levels, so that the cell is no longer DN. The levels of CD8 and CD4 expression are undetectable by direct cytofluorometric analysis (the cell continues to appear DN) but can easily be detected using panning techniques.[29,33,34] Most HSA^{+++} CD8^{lo}CD4^{lo}TCR^{lo} cells (85-95%) (Fig. 1) have completed the down-regulation of surface expression of IL-2R[29] and the remaining 5-15% still express low levels of IL-2R. The expression of CD8 and CD4 is dramatically enhanced if isolated CD8^{lo}CD4^{lo}TCR^{lo} IL-2R$^-$ thymocytes are cultured in simple medium overnight in the absence of thymic epithelium.[29,34] In contrast, HSA^{+++} IL-2R$^+$ DN cells do not express CD8 and CD4 when cultured under these conditions.[34] Therefore, CD8^{lo}CD4^{lo}TCR^{lo} thymocytes have obviously received signals that enable them to proceed autonomously to the CD8^{hi}CD4^{hi} double positive (DP) stage by an undefined mechanism.[35] These double positive immature thymocytes comprise approximately 80-85% of the total thymocyte number and are located in the thymic cortex. It is at this stage of development that selection (positive and negative) and intrathymic cell death takes place.

The CD3-TCR complex is expressed on CD8^{lo}CD4^{lo} thymocytes at 4- to 20-fold lower levels than in mature thymocytes. A substantial percentage (60-70%) of this population clearly stains positively with anti-CD3 monoclonal antibody.[29] At present it is not known whether the remaining cells in this population express extremely low levels of TCR, or whether they are actually TCR$^-$. While the αβ TCR heterodimer is coexpressed with CD3 on CD8^{lo}CD4^{lo} cells, no γδ TCR$^+$ cells have been detected in this population. Importantly, the expressed TCR is completely functional since the development of CD8^{lo}CD4^{lo} thymocytes can be impaired by treatment with immobilized anti-CD3 monoclonal antibody and hybridomas derived from CD8^{lo}CD4^{lo} cells can proliferate when TCR are crosslinked. This property renders the CD8^{lo}CD4^{lo} thymocytes susceptible to intrathymic selection from the moment they begin to express the TCR, although the chances of most thymocytes being selected at this stage are low due to the low density of the TCR and accessory molecules.

CD8^{lo}CD4^{lo} thymocytes can repopulate the irradiated thymus when injected intrathymically but cannot do so after intravenous injection[33] perhaps because they have lost the capacity to home to the thymus expressed by bone marrow precursors. After intrathymic transfer, the CD8^{lo}CD4^{lo} thymocytes will proliferate at least 15- to 20-fold.[33]

In B-cell development the expression of the immunoglobulin antigen receptor marks the end of proliferation[36] but the appearance of the TCR in the CD8^{lo}CD4^{lo} population correlates with the ability to proliferate. An alternative possibility is that the entire proliferative capacity of this subset resides in the TCR$^-$ population of CD8^{lo}CD4^{lo} cells. Direct labeling studies with monoclonal antibodies to the TCR and DNA proliferation markers (BUdR)[37,38] are necessary to distinguish between these alternatives. In general, the proliferative capacity of thymocytes decreases as they move from the more immature IL-2R[+] DN stage thymocytes to the CD8[hi]CD4[hi] stage, at which point all cell cycling ceases.[9,35,36]

Nakano et al[39] have described an IL-2R[-] DN thymocyte population that can become CD8[hi]CD4[hi] in vitro. Pearse et al[28] have also documented the presence of α4 TCR chain mRNA in the cytoplasm of HSA[+++,] IL-2R[-], Pgp-1[-] DN cells. Both these cell populations are equivalent to CD8[lo]CD4[lo]TCR[lo] cells. In fact, in the latter case the authors could actually detect by flow cytometry low levels of accessory molecules on these cells. Thereafter, when the extensive gene rearrangement and gene expression events are completed, the thymocytes begin intrathymic selection.

POSITIVE SELECTION

There are two categories of selection in the thymus: positive and negative.[40-45] Most researchers agree that these occur as separate and exclusive events and that the cells selecting thymocytes for positive and negative discrimination are not of the same type. During the process of selection, self-peptides bound to MHC class I and class II molecules on the surface of a selecting cell are recognized by TCR, CD8 and CD4 molecules on the differentiating thymocytes.

Cortical epithelial cells are the main cell type that mediates positive selection.[40,46,47] If the thymocyte TCR fits the MHC-peptide complex expressed by the cortical epithelium, it will be positively selected and escape cell death. It seems likely that the specificity of the TCR also dictates the CD8/CD4 phenotype of a developing T cell. If the receptor is specific for class I associated self-peptides, a thymocyte's CD8 molecule will corecognize a class I molecule, which will somehow fix the expression of CD8 and extinguish that of CD4. Likewise, a class II-associated peptide specificity of the TCR promotes a CD4[+]CD8[-] phenotype. As an alternative to this explanation, it is theoretically possible that the CD4/CD8 phenotype is fixed independently of the TCR specificity. In this model, to explain the bias of CD8[+] (or CD4[+]) thymocytes towards class I-restricted or class II-restricted antigen recognition, it is necessary to postulate that the maturation of a double positive thymocyte to become CD4[+]CD8[-] will have a nonproductive class I-specific TCR. Thus, one-half of all selection events would be nonproductive because of the mismatch between the TCR specificity and the fixation of accessory molecules. Although the first explanation is generally favored, there is yet no formal evidence to disprove the latter one.[49] What is almost certain however is that the selection process somehow prevents the programmed death of a thymocyte.

On the molecular level, the TCR presumably recognizes a complex of MHC-plus self peptide[49] in the same way that it recognizes MHC plus foreign peptide. Peptides contact the MHC by binding to one or more of the "pockets" in the MHC antigen-binding site.[40,41] A structural alteration to a critical pocket can abrogate binding of a given foreign[49] or self[49,50] peptide. This alteration can also abrogate the positive selection of the TCR repertoire specific for the same foreign peptide,[49] presumably by disrupting the binding (or changing the conformation) of self-peptides that mediate positive selection. For example, both ovalbumin peptide and self peptide that positively select α4 TCR repertoire specific for the ovalbumin peptide seem to bind to the same pocket of the MHC binding site. Binding to the same pocket could then be the mechanism for molecular mimicry. Experiments in TCR transgenic mice are consistent with the idea that self-peptides do participate in positive selection.[51,52] Although there is no definitive evidence as to which self-peptides guide the positive selection, or how diverse they may be, it is reasonable to assume that they can be derived by extracellular proteolysis of self proteins and by endogenous processing.[49]

NEGATIVE SELECTION AND A RECONCILIATION OF SELECTIONS

Negative selection, the process of clonal elimination of autoreactive thymocytes, is induced by hematopoietic and (probably) medullary epithelial cells.[40,46,47] Cell death induced by negative selection occurs by apoptosis (nonrandom programmed cell death) and the contact between the thymocyte and the cell mediating elimination again involves TCR, CD8 and CD4 molecules and MHC (class I or II) self-peptide complexes, respectively. However, negative selection does not necessarily involve the molecular contact identical to that occurring during positive selection. A double positive thymocyte can, for instance, be positively selected by TCR-CD8 interaction with an MHC class I-peptide complex but negatively selected by TCR-CD4 interaction with a MHC class II-peptide complex.

This leads to a major paradox in immunology: if both positive and negative selection involve the TCR recognition of self-MHC peptide complexes, how do any thymocytes avoid clonal elimination? This conundrum is far from being resolved, and there are numerous mutually nonexclusive theories to explain it. (An elegant discussion on how an unchanging receptor can induce different biological responses during T-cell ontogeny is presented by Finkel et al.[49]) Yet, if both positive and negative selection occur with the same set of ligands (self-peptides plus self-MHC molecules), then an affinity model may be more suitable to explain the controversy. In several recent publications,[49-52,55] it is proposed that the density of self-peptide MHC determinants required for positive selection is lower than the density necessary for intrathymic clonal elimination or peripheral activation. Self-peptides derived by extracellular and intracellular processing can mediate positive selection when bound to cortical epithelial cell MHC molecules. However, only a fraction of these peptides, predominantly the ones generated endogenously, would be present in concentrations high enough to induce intrathymic clonal elimination or clonal anergy. Also, the determinant density of most self-peptide MHC combinations would never be sufficient to activate the T cells in the periphery. In addition to selection via exogenous self-peptides, part of the repertoire could also be selected by unique, cortex specific peptide-MHC combinations[56,57] derived from endogenously generated determinants. However, the paucity of endogenously generated T-cell determinants,[58-60] makes it likely that their effect would be less significant than endogenous self-peptides.

The TCR repertoire generated according to this hypothesis would be diverse and innocuous under physiological conditions. Indeed, experimental evidence suggests that T cells reactive with extracellularly derived self-peptides normally exist without pathological consequences,[55] and they can only be activated by high (nonphysiological) concentrations of self-peptides.[55] Thus, some self-selected T cells are neither eliminated nor anergized and yet they are not autoaggressive under normal in vivo circumstances.

Although it is currently the prevailing opinion, it has not been definitively established that positive selection must precede negative selection. Indeed, recent studies describing the deletion of self-reactive thymocytes at an early double positive stage in TCR transgenic mice[43,43,61,62] seem to challenge this widely accepted view. The strength of contact between thymocytes and selecting cells depends on multivalent interactions between a number of molecules. The surface densities of these molecules and their affinity for their ligands, particularly the TCR affinity for peptide-MHC complex, are among the factors that determine the avidity of such contact. Thus, a given thymocyte can be positively or negatively selected as soon as (1) its avidity for a selecting cell reaches a certain threshold, (2) its TCR is structurally and biochemically coupled to signaling machinery and (3) the signaling machinery is completely assembled. This can occur at various stages of development, depending on the surface densities of TCR and accessory molecules on thymocytes, or on the particular peptide MHC determinant displayed by the selecting cell.

INTERMEDIATE STAGES: CD8^{hi} CD4^{lo}TCR^{lo} and CD8^{hi}CD4^{hi}TCR^{lo}

In principle, intrathymic selection can operate on a thymocyte as soon as the TCR is expressed on the surface, which is at the CD8^{lo}CD4^{lo}TCR^{lo} stage. However, the probability of selection increases with the increase of density of the TCR and accessory molecules. Within hours, CD8^{lo}CD4^{lo}TCR^{lo} cells upregulate their CD8 expression, so that an immature CD8^{hi}TCR^{lo} cell can readily be identified in mouse[63,64] and rat thymuses. In the mouse, these HSA^{+++}CD8^{hi}CD4^{lo}TCR^{lo} cells make up 30% of CD8^{hi} thymocytes, are immunologically competent,[64] can rapidly become CD8^{hi}CD4^{hi} in vitro,[20,65] and repopulate the irradiated thymus in vivo.[33] The conversion can be inhibited in vitro by cross-linking of the TCR on these cells with monoclonal antibody.[66]

It is quite possible that class I-restricted thymocytes can be selected to become CD8^{hi}CD4$^-$ at this stage rather than becoming CD8^{hi}CD4^{hi}. Selected cells would simply lose HSA and CD4, and gain higher levels of TCR. However, since the transition from the CD8^{hi}CD4^{lo}TCR^{lo} to the CD8^{hi}CD4^{hi}TCR^{lo} stage is completed within a few hours in vitro, and may be even faster in vivo, it seems probable that certain class I-restricted thymocytes will become CD8^{hi}CD4^{hi}TCR^{lo} before they get a chance to be positively selected and these cells then return to a CD8^{hi}CD4$^-$ phenotype after selection takes place. An additional factor limiting positive selection at the CD8^{hi}CD4^{lo} stage may be the availability of positively selecting MHC-peptide complexes.

Superficially, this latter view seems at odds with the prevailing view that CD8^{hi}CD4^{hi} thymocytes must be the exclusive direct precursors of mature single positive thymocytes, a hypothesis supported by two observations. First, single positive progeny can be obtained after the intrathymic transfer of CD8^{hi}CD4^{hi}TCR^{lo} blasts.[67] Second, certain self antigens, such as Mls^a and I-E are recognized by CD4^{hi} single positive T cells bearing TCR Vβ6 and Vβ17, respectively. When expressed intrathymically these antigens eliminate not only CD4[hi], but also CD8[hi] single positive cells bearing Vβ6 and Vβ17. [36,58] The CD8[hi] Vβ6[+] and Vβ17[+] cells can be rescued if the CD4 molecule is blocked by monoclonal antibodies during thymic development.[69,70] This suggests that all T cells have to pass through a CD8[hi]CD4[hi] stage. However, CD8[+]CD4[-] peripheral T cells bearing appropriate Vβ receptors have been shown to react with Mls[a] [71] or staphylococcal enterotoxins[72] plus-MHC class II molecules in the apparent absence of CD4. This may mean that, in certain cases, the TCR alone can be subject to deletion, irrespective of accessory molecules. Since immature CD8[hi] thymocytes are CD4[lo], it is quite possible that even these low levels of CD4 are sufficient to enhance the avidity of Vβ6 or Vβ17 bearing CD8 thymocytes for the MHC class II-Mls molecular complex on the eliminating cells. Consequently, CD4 blocking could allow the appearance of CD8 cells bearing the forbidden Vβ product.

The results of intrathymic transfer of CD8[hi]CD4[hi] thymocyte blasts[67] actually lend support to the hypothesis that after transfer, CD8[+] single positive cells appear significantly later than CD4[+] single positive cells. This result can be interpreted as a consequence of selection-mediated depletion of class I restricted cells from CD8[hi]CD4[hi] thymocytes. Additional experiments are in progress to document the existence of positive selection at a CD8[hi]CD4[lo] level.

HSA[+++]CD8[hi]CD4[hi]CD3[hi] thymocytes are the next stage in the life of a thymocyte. These cells constitute up to 85% of all thymocytes and are immunocompetent but at least 95% of them will never reach the peripheral circulation. The selection processes extensively operate on this subset of precursors of single positive cells.[67] When the CD8[hi]CD4[hi] thymocyte gets positively selected, one of its accessory molecules is downregulated. HSA expression will also decrease, and the expression of TCR will increase (Fig. 1). CD8[hi]CD4[lo]CD3[lo] thymocytes have a very low proliferative capacity in vivo and CD8[hi]CD4[hi]CD3[lo] thymocytes proliferate even less, if at all.[36]

FINAL MATURATION: SINGLE POSITIVE THYMOCYTES AND THEIR IMMEDIATE PRECURSORS

After positive selection, TCR expression gradually reaches mature levels. Class I restricted thymocytes have TCR and CD8 that corecognize self-peptide-MHC class I complexes and will down-regulate the CD4 molecule. The opposite will happen in successfully selected class II restricted CD8[hi]CD4[hi] thymocytes. The final maturation is gradual and slow, involving numerous changes. At first it is hard to distinguish phenotypically positively selected CD8[hi] cells that down-regulate CD4 from immature CD8[hi] cells that acquire high levels of CD4. Eventually, the difference becomes more obvious, with the loss of the HSA and the expression of higher levels of TCR typical of a selected thymocyte. Finally, the Qa-2 molecule (an additional murine MHC Class I molecule whose function is unknown) is expressed by mature thymocytes (Fig. 1).[3]

It is much easier to follow the selected CD4[hi] thymocytes. It is possible to isolate two subsets of CD4[hi] single positive thymocytes from H-2[b] mice.[73] The precise phenotype of these cells is HSA[+++]CD8[lo]CD4[hi]CD3[hi] and HSA[+/-]CD8[-]CD4[hi]CD3[hi], their numerical ratio is 2:1 and differences in functional reactivity can be detected between the two subsets. The CD8[-] subset could autonomously proliferate in response to alloantigens, whereas the CD8^{lo} subset requires exogenous IL-2.[73] Whether the CD8^{lo}CD4^{hi}CD3^{hi} thymocytes can be tolerized, activated or induced to die under in vivo conditions is an open question. It is not certain whether full maturation (including the acquisition of IL-2 secreting phenotype) has to be completed intrathymically. Research on peripheral T-cell maturation will undoubtedly yield useful information on the subject.

REFERENCES

1. Miller JFAP, Osoba D. Current concepts of the immunologic function of the thymus. Physiol Rev 1967; 47: 437-520.

2. Owen JJT, Ritter M. Tissue interaction in the development of thymus lymphocytes. J Exp Med 1969; 129: 431-34.

3. Fowlkes BJ, Pardoll DM. Molecular and cellular events of T-cell development. Adv Immunol 1989; 44: 207-64.

4. von Boehmer H. The developmental biology of T lymphocytes. Ann Rev Immunol 1988; 6: 309-35.

5. Fowlkes BJ, Edison L, Mathieson BJ, Chused TM. Early T lymphocytes. Differentiation in vivo of adult intrathymic precursor cells. J Exp Med 1985; 162: 802-06.

6. Budd RC, Miescher GC, Howe RC, et al. Developmentally regulated expression of T-cell receptor β chain variable domains in immature thymocytes. J Exp Med 1987; 166: 577-82.

7. Lesley J, Shulte R, Hyman R. Kinetics of thymus repopulation by intrathymic progenitors after intravenous injection: Evidence for successive repopulation by an IL-2R$^+$, Pgp-1$^-$ and by an IL-2R$^-$, Pgp-1$^+$ progenitor. Cell Immunol 1988; 177: 378-88.

8. Howe RC, MacDonald HR. Heterogeneity of immature (Lyt2$^-$/L3T4$^-$) thymocytes: Identification of four major phenotypically distinct subsets differing in cell cycle status and in vitro activation requirements. J Immunol 1988; 140: 1047-52.

9. Ewing T, Egerton M, Wilson A, et al. Subpopulations of CD4$^-$CD8$^-$ murine thymocytes: Differences in proliferation rates in vivo and proliferative responses in vitro. Eur J Immunol 1988; 18: 261-68.

10. Fowlkes BJ, Kruisbeek AM, Ton-That H, et al. A novel population of T-cell receptor αβ bearing thymocytes which predominantly expresses a single Vβ gene family. Nature 1987; 329: 251-54.

11. Havran WL, Allison JP. Developmentally ordered appearance of thymocytes expressing different T-cell antigen receptors. Nature 1988; 335: 443-45.

12. Lew AM, Pardoll DM, Maloy WL, et al. Characterization of T-cell receptor gamma chain expression in a subset of murine thymocytes. Science 1986; 234: 1401-05.

13. Husmann LA, Shimonkevitz RP, Crispe IN, et al. Thymocyte subpopulations during early fetal development in the BALB/c mouse. J Immunol 1988; 141: 736-40.

14. Crispe IN, Moore MW, Husmann LA, et al. Differentiation potential of subsets of CD4$^-$8$^-$ thymocytes. Nature 1987; 329: 251-54.

15. Shimonkevitz RP, Husmann LA, Bevan MJ, et al. Transient expression of IL-2 receptor precedes the differentiation of immature thymocytes. Nature 1987; 329: 157-59.

16. Scollay R, Shortman K. Identification of early stages of T lymphocyte development in the thymic cortex and medulla. J Immunol 1985; 134: 3632-42.

17. Wilson A, D'Amico A, Ewing T, et al. Subpopulations of early thymocytes: A cross-correlation flow cytometric analysis of adult Lyt2⁻ L3T4⁻ (CD8⁻ CD4) thymocytes using eight different surface markers. J Immunol 1988; 140: 1461-69.

18. Russel JH, Meleedy-Rey P, McCulley DE, et al. Evidence for CD8⁻ independent T-cell maturation in transgenic mice. J Immunol 1990; 144: 3318-25.

19. Hugo P, Waanders GA, Scollay R, Petrie HT, Boyd RL. Characterization of immature CD4⁺8⁻3⁻thymocytes. Eur J Immunol 1991; 21: 835-41.

20. MacDonald HR, Budd RC, Howe RC. A CD3⁻ subset of CD8⁺ cell. Eur J Immunol 1988; 18: 519-23.

21. Paterson DJ, Williams AF. An intermediate cell in thymocyte differentiation that expresses CD8 but not CD4 antigen. J Exp Med 1987; 166: 1603-08.

22. Shortman K, Wilson A, Egerton M, Pearse M, Scollay R. Immature CD4⁻ CD8⁺ murine thymocytes. Cell Immunol 1988; 113: 462-68.

23. MacDonald HR, Howe RC, Pedrazzini T, et al. T-cell lineages repertoire selection and tolerance induction. Immunol Rev 1988; 104: 157-79.

24. Yankelevich B, Knoblock C, Nowicki M, et al. A novel cell type responsible for marrow graft rejection in mice: T cells with NK phenotype cause acute rejection of marrow grafts. J Immunol 1989; 142: 3423-30.

25. Ballas ZK, Rasmunssen W. NK1.1⁺ thymocytes: Adult murine CD4⁻, CD8⁻ thymocytes contain an NK1.1⁺, CD3⁺, CD5ʰⁱ, CD44ʰⁱ, TCR⁻VB8⁺ subset. J Immunol 1990; 145: 1039-45.

26. Hyman R, Lesley J, Schulte R, et al. Progenitor cells in the thymus: Most thymus-homing progenitor cells in the adult mouse thymus bear Pgp-1 glycoprotein but not interleukin-2 receptor on their surface. Cell Immunol 1986; 101: 320-24.

27. Lesley J, Hyman R, Schulte R. Evidence that the Pgp-1 glycoprotein is expressed on thymus-homing progenitor cells in the thymus. Cell Immunol 1985; 91: 397-402.

28. Pearse M, Wu L, Egerton M, et al. A murine early thymocyte developmental sequence is marked by transient expression of the interleukin 2 receptor. Proc Natl Acad Sci USA 1989; 86: 1614-18.

29. Nikolic-Zugic J, Moore MW. T-cell receptor expression on immature thymocytes with in vivo and in vitro precursor potentials. Eur J Immunol 1989; 19: 1957-60.

30. Ceredig R, Lowenthal JW, Nabholtz M, et al. Expression of Interleukin-2 receptors as a differentiation marker of intrathymic stem cells. Nature 1985; 314: 98-100.

31. Raulet DH. Expression and function of interleukin-2 receptors on immature thymocytes. Nature 1985; 314: 101-03.

32. Habu S, Okumara S, Diamanstein T, et al. Expression of interleukin-2 receptor on murine fetal thymocytes. Eur. J. Immunol. 1985; 15: 456-60.

33. Nikolic-Zugic J, Bevan MJ. Thymocytes expressing CD8 differentiate into CD4⁺ cells following intrathymic injection. Proc Natl Acad Sci USA 1988; 85: 8633-37.

34. Nikolic-Zugic J, Moore MW, Bevan MJ. Characterization of the subset of immature thymocytes which can undergo rapid in vitro differentiation. Eur J Immunol 1989; 19: 649-53.

35. Clevers H, Owen MJ. Towards a molecular understanding of T-cell differentiation. Immunol Today 1991; 12: 86-92.

36. Osmond DG, Owen JJT. Pre-B cells in bone marrow: size distribution profile, proliferative capacity and peanut agglutinin binding of cytoplasmic *u* chain-bearing cell population in normal and regenerating bone marrow. Immunology 1984; 51: 333-39.

37. Penit C. In vivo thymocyte maturation: BUdR labeling of cycling thymocytes and phenotypic analysis of their progeny support the signal lineage model. J Immunol 1986; 137: 2115-21.

38. Penit C, Vasseur F. Sequential events in thymocyte differentiation and thymic regeneration revealed by a combination of bromodeoxyuridine DNA labeling and antimitotic drug treatment. J Immunol 1988; 140: 3315-23.

39. Nakano N, Hardy RR, Kishimoto T. Identification of intrathymic T progenitor cells by expression of Thy-1, IL-2 receptor and CD3. Eur J Immunol 1987; 17: 1567-71.

40. Sprent J, Lo D, Gao KK, Ron Y. T-cell selection in the thymus. Immunol Rev 1988; 101: 173-90.

41. Bevan MJ. In a radiation chimera, host H-2 antigens determine immune responsiveness of donor cytotoxic cells. Nature 1977; 269: 417-18.

42. Kisielow P, Teh HS, Bluthmann H, et al. Positive selection of antigen-specific T cells in thymus by restricting MHC molecules. Nature 1988; 335: 730-33.

43. Sha WC, Nelson CA, Newberry RD, et al. Selective expression of an antigen receptor on CD8⁻bearing T lymphocytes in transgenic mice. Nature 1988; 335: 271-74.

44. Teh HS, Kisielow P, Scott B, et al. Thymic major histocompatibility complex antigens and the a β T-cell receptor determine the CD4/CD8 phenotype of T cells. Nature 1988; 335: 229-33.

45. Kappler JW, Roehm N, Marrack P. T-cell tolerance by clonal elimination in the thymus. Cell 1987; 49: 273-80.

46. Lo D, Sprent J. Identity of cells that imprint H-2-restricted T-cell specificity in the thymus. Nature 1986; 319: 672-75.

47. Benoist C, Mathis D. Positive selection of the T-cell repertoire: Where and when does it occur? Cell 1989; 58: 1027-33.

48. Finkel TH, Kubo RT, Cambier JC. T-cell development and transmembrane signaling: Changing biological responses through an unchanging receptor. Immunol Today 1990; 12: 79-85.

49. Nikolic-Zugic J, Bevan MJ. Role of self-peptides in positively selecting the T-cell repertoire. Nature 1990; 344: 65-67.

50. Garrett TPJ, Saper MA, Bjorkman PJ, et al. Specificity pockets for the side chains of peptide antigens in HLA-Aw68. Nature 1989; 342: 692-96.

51. Sha WC, Nelson CA, Newberry RD, et al. Positive selection of transgenic receptor-bearing thymocytes by K^b antigen is altered by K^b mutations that involve peptide binding. Proc Natl Acad Sci USA 1990; 87: 6186-90.

52. Berg LJ, Frank GD, Davis MM. The effects of MHC gene dosage and allelic variation on T-cell receptor selection. Cell 1990; 60: 1043-53.

53. Keer JF, Wyllie AH, Currie AR. Apoptosis: A basic biological phenomenon with wide-ranging implications in tissue kinetics. Br J Cancer 1972; 26: 239-57.

54. Smith CA, Williams GT, Kingston R, et al. Antibodies to CD3/T-cell receptor complex induce death by apoptosis in immature T cells in thymic cultures. Nature 1989; 337: 181-84.

55. Schild H, Rotzchke O, Kalbacher H, et al. Limit of T-cell tolerance to self proteins by peptide presentation. Science 1989; 247: 1587-89.

56. Marrack P, Kappler J. The T-cell repertoire for antigen and MHC. Immnuol Today 1988; 9: 308-15.

57. Kourilsky P, Claverie JM. MHC restriction, alloreactivity, and thymic education: A common link? Cell 1989; 56: 327-29.

58. Carbone FR, Moore MW, Sheil MJ, et al. Induction of cytotoxic T lymphocytes by primary in vitro stimulation with peptides. J Exp Med 1988; 167: 1767-79.

59. Moore MW, Carbone FR, Bevan MJ. Introduction of soluble protein into the class I pathway of antigen processing and presentation. Cell 1988; 54: 777-85.

60. Townsend A, Bodmer H. Antigen recognition by class I-restricted T lymphocytes. Annu Rev Immunol 1989; 7: 601-24.

61. Berg LJ, Fazekas de St. Groth B, Pullen AM, et al. Phenotypic differences between αβ versus β T-cell receptor transgenic mice undergoing negative selection. Nature 1989; 340: 559-62.

62. Pircher H, Burki K, Lang R, et al. Tolerance induction in double specific T-cell receptor transgenic mice varies with antigen. Nature 1989; 342: 559-61.

63. Bluestone JA, Pardoll DM, Sharrow SO, et al. Characterization of murine thymocytes with CD3 associated T-cell receptor structures. Nature 1987; 326: 82-84.

64. Crispe IN, Bevan MJ. Expression and functional significance of the J1.1d marker on mouse thymocytes. J Immunol 1987; 138: 2013-18.

65. Paterson DJ, Williams AF. An intermediate cell in thymocyte differentiation that expresses CD8 but not CD4 antigen. J Exp Med 1987; 166: 1603-08.

66. Hunig T. Cross-linking of the T-cell antigen receptor interferes with the generation of CD4$^+$8$^+$ thymocytes from their immediate CD4$^-$8$^+$ precursors. Eur J Immunol 1988; 18: 2089-92.

67. Guidos CJ, Weissman IL, Adkins B. Intrathymic maturation of murine T lymphocytes from CD8$^+$ precursors. Proc Natl Acad Sci USA 1989; 86: 7542-46.

68. MacDonald HR, Schneider R, Lees RK, et al. T-cell receptor Vβ use predicts reactivity and tolerance to Mls^a-encoded antigens. Nature 1988; 332: 40-45.

69. Fowlkes BJ, Schwartz RH, Pardoll DM. Deletion of self-reactive thymocytes occurs at a CD4$^+$8$^+$ precursor stage. Nature 1988; 334: 620-23.

70. MacDonald HR, Hengartner H, Pedrazzini T. Intrathymic deletion of self-reactive cells prevented by neonatal anti-CD4 antibody treatment. Nature 1988; 335: 174-76.

71. Webb SR, Sprent J. Response of mature unprimed CD8$^+$ T cells in Mls^a determinants. J Exp Med 1990; 171: 953-58.

72. Callahan J, Herman A, Kappler JW, et al. Stimulation of B10.BR T cells with superantigenic Staphylococcal toxins. J Immunol 1990; 144: 2473-79.

73. Nikolic-Zugic J, Bevan MJ. Functional and phenotypic delineation of two subsets of CD4 single positive cells in the thymus. Int Immunol 1990; 2: 135-41.

CHAPTER 9

T-CELL ANTIGEN RECEPTOR

Antigen specific responses have historically been divided into humoral immunity and cell-mediated immunity based on the ability to transfer specific protection, or passively immunize, with either serum or cells respectively. Humoral immunity was shown to be mediated by antibody molecules in a long series of investigations starting with the demonstration of serum substances that would transfer protection to bacterial toxins in the 19th century and culminating in the 1960s with the work of Edelman and Porter on the structure of antibody molecules found in serum and those secreted from human and mouse plasmacytomas.[1-3] The reaction resulting from cell-mediated immunity was first described by Edward Jenner in the last part of the 18th century in his studies on the immunity to cowpox. In these studies, he noted that a local reaction developed after 24 to 48 hours at a site of reinoculation of a previously immunized individual. Experiments by Landsteiner and Chase in 1942 showed that this type of immunity, referred to as delayed-type hypersensitivity (DTH), could be transferred by cells but not serum, and was specific for the immunizing antigen.[4] A related form of immunity, namely allograft rejection, was elucidated in a long series of studies directed at an understanding of the genetics of transplant rejection. Mitchison showed that this type of immunity was also transferred with cells.[5]

The form of antigen recognized by T cells is entirely different from that recognized by antibodies or by B cells bearing a membrane form of antibody as a receptor. Gell and Benacerraf showed in 1957 that antisera produced against a series of proteins were specific for the native protein, whereas a DTH response could be elicited equally well by reinoculation with either the denatured or native forms.[6] In addition, there is an essential difference between the forms of antigen recognized by T cells and antibodies. Whereas antibodies bind antigen in solution, T cells only recognize antigen bound to another cell. In fact, the landmark work of Zinkernagel and Doherty in 1974 demonstrated that T cells recognize antigen determinants in association with determinants present on major histocompatibility complex (MHC) molecules.[7] This topic is essential to the understanding of cell interactions in the immune system.

GENETIC ORGANIZATION OF THE GENES ENCODING THE T-CELL RECEPTOR

α Chain

There is a single α chain C-region in humans and mice (Fig. 1) [composed of four exons encoding (a) the constant region domain, (b) 16 amino acids including the cysteine that forms the interchain disulfide bond, (c) the transmembrane and intracytoplasmic domains, and (d) the 3' untranslated region[8]]. There are a large number of J-regions upstream of the C-region (estimated from frequency of usage to be approximately 50).[9] This gene organization was determined from direct mapping of overlapping DNA fragments cloned into lambda phage or cosmid vectors.[10] These clones were isolated by "chromosome walking" in which one end of a DNA fragment was used as a probe to isolate another overlapping clone, and the other end of the second clone was used as a probe to isolate a third clone, and so on. The overlapping clones were mapped for the presence of the C-region exons and the various known J-regions. Some of the coding sequences were completely sequenced and although only the organization of the mouse α locus is completely known, information thus far available indicates that the organization of the human α chain locus is essentially the same.[11]

An undetermined distance upstream of the Jα gene elements are located Vα gene elements (Fig. 1), and a mature, transcribable gene is formed by the rearrangement and apposition of a Vα segment and a Jα segment (Fig. 2). For α chains the mechanism of rearrangement appears to be a deletion of the sequences between the V-region and J-region (Fig. 2a).[11] The α chain V-regions are present as cross-hybridizing gene families consisting of 3 to 20 members.[114] Thus far there have been 13 families identified in the mouse and there is likely to be roughly equivalent number in humans. An important contribution to the diversity of the α chain is the "combinatorial joining"

Fig. 1. Organization of the gene elements encoding the T-cell receptor α and δ chain loci. [From Hedrick SM. T lymphocyte receptors. In: Paul WE, ed. Fundamental Immunology, 2nd ed. New York: Raven Press, 1989.]

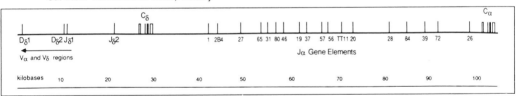

Fig. 2. Schematic diagram showing the mechanisms of gene rearrangements. [From Hedrick SM. T lymphocyte receptors. In: Paul WE, ed. Fundamental Immunology, 2nd ed. New York: Raven Press, 1989.]

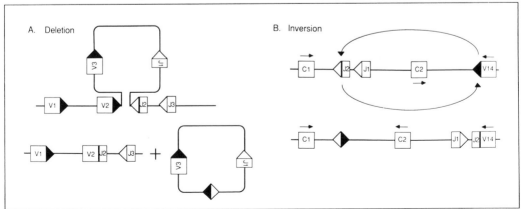

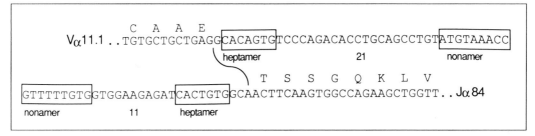

Fig. 3. Rearrangement and junctional diversity of α chain V and J-regions. [From Hedrick SM. T lymphocyte receptors. In: Paul WE, ed. Fundamental Immunology, 2nd ed. New York: Raven Press, 1989.]

of different V-regions and J-regions. If the V-regions number 100 and the J-regions 50, then the total number of V-J combinations is on the order of 5000 α chains.

Downstream of the germline α chain V-region there is a canonical heptamer-nonamer sequence consisting of a conserved 7 nucleotides and 9 nucleotides separated by a spacer of 21 nucleotides (Fig. 3). The sequence downstream of the V-region in immunoglobulins is typically CACAGTG-[22 nucleotides]-ACAAAAACC. Upstream of the germline α chain J-region is a nonamer-heptamer sequence separated by 11 nucleotides. The J-region sequence in immunoglobulins is typically the inverse of the V-region or GGTTTTTGT-[12 nucleotides]-CACTGTG.[12] Since the TCR α chain and immunoglobulin heavy chain sequences are interchangeable, in certain human diseases, V-region genes from the immunoglobulin heavy chain locus can rearrange with J-region genes from the TCR α chain locus to form a hybrid TCR Vα-Ig J$_H$ rearranged gene.[12]

An additional mechanism for the generation of diversity is the sequence variability at the junction of the V-region and the J-region. The rearranged genes have sequences contributed from the V-region and the J-region, and in addition, there are often nucleotides that were not present in the germline. These nontemplate-dependent sequences have been found in immunoglobulin heavy chain genes and are termed N-regions.[13] They presumably originate from the random addition of nucleotides during the rearrangement event, perhaps catalyzed by an enzyme similar or identical to an enzyme, 3' deoxynucleotidyl terminal transferase, found in the thymus and other tissues.[13] Although there are N-region nucleotides in immunoglobulin heavy chain genes that result from V-D-J rearrangements, light chain genes that result from V-J rearrangements do not have N-region nucleotides. The α chain genes are, therefore, analogous to immunoglobulin light chains with respect to the number of genetic elements involved in rearrangements, but dissimilar in terms of the contribution of N-regions.

β Chain

There are two β chain constant region genes in all species thus far analyzed and they are tandemly arranged (Fig. 4).[14,15] In the mouse, these two β chain C-regions differ by only four conserved amino acid substitutions, and there is no known functional difference between the two. They are used interchangeably in all types of T cells, even among those with essentially the same antigen specificity and surface phenotype.[16] Thus these β chain isotypes are not analogous to immunoglobulin isotypes in which differences in C-regions specify antibodies with different functions. Thus, the need for selection for two C-regions is thus not clear. It has been suggested that the two β chain regions allow for more J-regions, but considering the organization of the α chain locus, there is no constraint on the number of upstream J-regions that can be associated with a single C-region. The only exception to this β chain gene organization known thus far is in New Zealand white (NZW) mice.[17,18] There is a deletion in the NZW mouse β chain region that spans the Cβ1 and the Jβ2 loci such that transcription originating with a Vβ-Jβ1 exon includes the adjacent Cβ2 (Fig. 4). Although there is no known effect of this deletion, interestingly, (NZW x NZB)F₁ mice have a high propensity for developing autoimmunity.

Each of the β chain constant genes consists of four exons encoding (a) the constant region domain, (b) six amino acids including the cysteine involved in the interchain disulfide bond, (c) the membrane spanning domain, and (d) the cytoplasmic domain and the 3' untranslated region. Upstream of each C-region are seven J-regions and one D-region. In the mouse, there is one pseudogene in each cluster. The Dβ1 gene can rearrange with all 12 functional J-regions, whereas Dβ2 can rearrange only with Jβ2.1-Jβ2.7.

The order of rearrangements of the β chain locus is the same as that of the immunoglobulin heavy chain locus. The first rearrangement events involve D joining to J with the deletion of the sequences separating the gene elements (Fig. 2a). This can occur on both chromosomes and for both Dβ1 and Dβ2 sequentially, thus resulting in from one to four D-J rearrangement events in each T-cell. The second type of rearrangement involves a V to D joining. The probability of maintaining the proper reading frame from the V-region through the rearrangement junction into the J-region is one out of three.[11] With a probability of 2 out of 3, the genes do not maintain the proper reading frame and produce a frame shift product. Although the regulation of rearrangements in T cells is not well worked out, the evidence indicates that the presence of an intact β chain polypeptide suppresses further V-region rearrangements.[19]

Nucleotides that are not specified in the germline genes, i.e., N-regions, are located between the V, D, and J-regions. The rearrangement signals downstream of the V-region consist of a heptamer-23 nucleotide-nonamer sequence similar to that found in immunoglobulin V-regions. The D-region

Fig. 4. β chain constant region locus. Organization of the D, J and C-region gene elements encoding the β chain. [From Hedrick SM. T lymphocyte receptors. In: Paul WE, ed. Fundamental Immunology, 2nd ed. New York: Raven Press, 1989.]

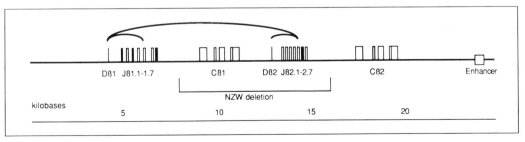

has the corresponding rearrangement sequences, nonamer-12 nucleotide-heptamer upstream of the coding region and heptamer-23 nucleotide-nonamer downstream. Upstream of the J-region the rearrangement signal is nonamer-12 nucleotide-heptamer. From the rules governing immunoglobulin rearrangements, namely, the "12-23 rule," gene elements flanked by a 23-nucleotide spacer can only rearrange to those flanked by a 12-nucleotide spacer, and vice versa. For immunoglobulin heavy chain genes, this rule implies that V-regions can only rearrange with D-regions; however, an inspection of the β chain genes indicates that the V-region could, in principle, rearrange to either a D-region or directly to a J-region. In fact, an analysis of the β chain sequences from antigen specific T cells indicates that the absence of a contribution from the D-region is extremely rare.

For most of the V-regions, gene rearrangement involves simple sequence deletion.[13,14] For all the V-regions identified upstream of the constant regions, the rearrangement occurs via deletion (Fig. 2a) since the genes are in the same transcriptional orientation as the D and J gene elements. However, Vβ14 in the mouse is downstream of the C-regions and in the opposite orientation. Rearrangements involving Vβ14 occur via inversion (Fig. 2b) without the loss of the sequences separating the V and J-regions.[22] All these mechanisms of rearrangement do occur based on an analysis of the genetic organization of the β chain locus in mature T-cell clones.[23] In fact, the products of rearrangement by deletion have been isolated, namely, closed circles of DNA containing sequences originating from the chromosomal DNA between D and J-regions.[24]

A structural map of the human and mouse Vβ gene elements has been determined by a combination of molecular techniques.[20,21] Much of the data was derived by direct mapping of overlapping cloned DNA as described for the mapping of J-regions in the α chain locus. A second technique for identifying the order of V-regions involves deletional mapping studies. This technique takes advantage of the fact that the rearrangement of a V-region and D-region deletes the DNA located between these two genetic elements. In principle, in a murine T-cell that has rearranged Vβ1 to Dβ1, the V-region located between the two genetic elements are deleted from the chromosome. This can be seen by genomic Southern blotting with the caveat that the paired chromosome also contributes an allele. Therefore, T-cell clones that have V-regions rearranged on both chromosomes must be analyzed. A third technique is to analyze the chromosomal organization directly by genomic Southern blotting. The limitation of this technique is that conventional agarose gel electrophoresis can only resolve restriction fragments less than approximately 20-30 kilobases. This will include most restriction fragments generated by endonucleases that recognize a six-base sequence. However, many V-regions are separated by more than 20 kilobases and thus cannot be mapped with respect to one another using this technique.

The human and murine β chain loci are similar in organization. Of interest is the fact that many of the V-regions in the mouse have a direct homolog in the human. This indicates that most of the evolutionary divergence of the V-regions occurred before human-mouse speciation, and although the human V-regions have expanded by duplication to a somewhat greater extent than those in the mouse, the V-regions have remained largely conserved. The possibility that at least some of the V-regions confer a survival advantage is suggested by these data.

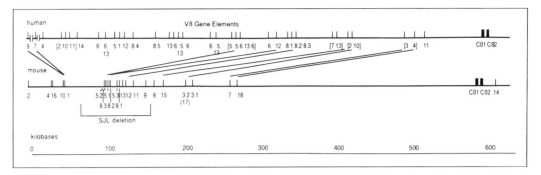

Fig. 5. Organization of the entire T-cell receptor β chain locus. [From Hedrick SM. T lymphocyte receptors. In: Paul WE, ed. Fundamental Immunology, 2nd ed. New York: Raven Press, 1989.]

The organization of the β chain genes is relatively conserved between laboratory strains of mice such that there are few restriction fragment length polymorphisms. For example, there has been identified an allelic variation in SJL, C57BR, C57L, and related strains of mice (Fig. 5). These three strains of mice have a deletion in the V-region locus including Vβ5.2-Vβ9. Since this region includes the Vβ8 family, T cells from these mice fail to react with the monoclonal antibodies KJ16 (that recognizes Vβ8.1 and Vβ8.2), F23.2 (recognizes Vβ8.2), and F23.1 (recognizes Vβ8.1, Vβ8.2, and Vβ8.3).[25] In addition, these three mice express a V-region, Vβ17, that is not expressed in other strains of mice. The monoclonal antibody KJ23 recognizes receptors containing Vβ17 and thus all laboratory mouse strains are negative for KJ23 with the exception of SJL, C57BR and C57L mice.[26]

γ Chain

The human V-region organization consists of at least 14 genes in a tandem array, and each is potentially capable of rearranging to any five J-regions (Fig. 6).[27-30] Six of the V-regions are pseudogenes. The two C-region genes in the human differ in that Cγ2 contains two to three duplicated second exons that have lost the cysteine residue involved in the interchain disulfide bond. Thus Cγ2 bearing human T cells have an extra large γ-chain that is not disulfide bonded to its δ chain partner. In contrast, all three functional γ chain C-regions in the mouse are homologous to the human Cγ1 gene, and thus mouse γ chains are always of 30,000 to 40,000 MW and disulfide bonded to a δ chain. Human γ chains can range from 35,000 to 55,000 MW with the larger ones noncovalently associated with a δ chain. The organization in the mouse is different from the human in that there are three separate rearranging loci.[27,31] The nomenclature used to identify the V, J, and C-regions is adopted from Garman et al.[31]

In comparing the homologies between the human and the mouse V-region genes (Fig. 6), the human Vγ8 and Vγ11 are more homologous to the mouse Vγ5 and Vγ1.1, respectively, than to any other human Vγ genes. This reinforces the concept, once again, that the diversity of the V-regions occurred to some extent before human-mouse speciation.

Analogous to the α chain and immunoglobulin light chains, the γ chain gene results from a single V- to J-region rearrangement. The V-regions each

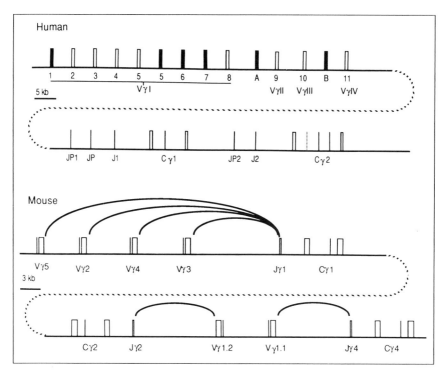

Fig. 6. Organization of the γ chain locus. [From Hedrick SM. T lymphocyte receptors. In: Paul WE, ed. Fundamental Immunology, 2nd ed. New York: Raven Press, 1989.]

have a heptamer-23 nucleotide-nonamer sequence downstream of the coding region, and the J-regions have a nonamer-12 nucleotide-heptamer upstream of the coding region. Similar to α chains, N-region nucleotides added between the V and J-regions are common and range from 0 to 14 nucleotides.

δ Chain

The δ chain D-, J-, and C-region gene elements are located within the α chain gene locus between the Vα and Jα genes in both humans and mice (Fig. 1).[32] There is a single Cδ-region gene composed of four exons, and upstream there have been found, thus far, two Jδ regions and two Dδ regions. Thus, in the three principal types of receptors in the immune system encoded by rearranging genes, there is a symmetry. In each case one of the genes is formed by a V-J rearrangement (immunoglobulin light chains, TCR α chain, TCR γ chain) and the other is formed by a V-D-J rearrangement (immunoglobulin heavy chain, TCR β chain, TCR δ chain).

T-Cell Antigen Receptor Maturation: VDJ Gene Segment Recombination

The ability of T lymphocyte receptor V, D and J gene segments to rearrange generates much of the receptor diversity that is the hallmark of the immune system. The mechanism of VDJ recombination and the manner in which this site-specific recombination activity is controlled has remained a difficult topic to study. The major difficulty stems from the inability to identify the components of VDJ recombination and to reproduce this re-action in a cell-free system. Likewise, the nature of elements that control the tissue and stage specificity of the reaction has remained somewhat controversial, primarily because of the paucity of readily manipulable systems that allow the normal physiological constraints on this activity to be unequivocally identified. Lately, however, there have been significant advances in both of these areas that may allow detailed resolution of the VDJ recombination process.

ACTIVITIES INVOLVED IN VDJ RECOMBINATION

General Mechanism

The VDJ recombination process is a complex reaction that involves numerous components, many of which have yet to be clearly identified. Much of what is known about the mechanistic details has been derived from analyses of the substrates and products of the reaction.[33] In fact, there has been little change in our overall view of the recombination process during the past 10 years.[13,34] Several lines of evidence indicate that the VDJ recombination reaction is carried out by the same processes (referred to as VDJ recombinase) for all the different families of immunoglobulin (Ig) and T-cell receptor (TCR) variable region gene segments.[35] Put simply, the mechanism involves recognition of conserved heptamer-spacer-nonamer sequence elements that flank each germ-line V, D and J segment, the introduction of double-strand breaks between the elements to be joined and the flanking RS sequences, potential loss and/or addition of nucleotides at the coding junctions, and the polymerization and ligation activities to complete the joining process (Fig. 2a).[13]

The existence of specific mechanisms to delete or add nucleotides at coding junctions appears to have evolved as a way to promote sequence diversity in the portion of the Ig or TCR proteins encoded by these junctional regions.[33] One long noted aspect of this site-specific reaction is the different handling of the coding and RS joins[34,35] in that the latter rarely involve nucleotide deletions.[36] Analyses of the mouse severe combined immunodeficiency (*scid*) mutation have reinforced this observation.[34,35] The development of novel transient recombination substrates to analyze efficiently the products of large numbers of substrate joins[37] and the use of the polymerase chain reaction (PCR) to analyze large numbers of endogenous coding joins[38] have led to further insights into the VDJ recombination mechanism,[34] including the generation of P elements (small duplications) at coding joins.[38]

The RS sequences that flank V, D and J-segments are sufficient to target the site-specific activities of the VDJ recombination system to the adjacent coding sequence.[39,40] It was postulated that such recognition was followed by the introduction of double-strand breaks in the DNA precisely at these junctures.[13] Although the exact form of such breaks remains to be determined, their existence has been unequivocally demonstrated.[41] The relative orientation of the involved sequences in the chromosone determines the fate of the reaction products. If two sequences are in "opposite" transcriptional orientation, the reaction will lead to inversion of the segment of DNA between the coding and RS joins with retention of all products in the chromosome (Fig. 2b). If the two sequences are in the same transcriptional orientation, the coding joins will be retained in the chromosome while the

RS joins will be deleted as a circle. The identification of these circular products has been reported[42,24] although linear (unligated) deletion products have also observed to accumulate in the thymus.[41] VDJ recombination substrates, designed to study aspects of the joining process following transfection into cells, have exploited both the inversional and deletional modes of this reaction.[35,43]

ESSENTIAL TISSUE-SPECIFIC COMPONENTS

By analogy to other site-specific recombination systems, specificity for the VDJ reaction could be orchestrated by one or two specific gene products while other events (for example, ligation) might be effected by ubiquitous cellular activities recruited to carry out their functions in the context of VDJ recombination.[44] Recently, two genes have been identified that, when expressed simultaneously, are sufficient to generate VDJ recombinase activity in all cell types examined.[45,46] These two genes were designated "recombinase activation genes"—RAG-1 and RAG-2. The nonspecific name stemmed from the fact that it was not (and has not yet been) possible to determine unequivocally whether these genes encode the tissue-specific components of VDJ recombinase; it remains possible that one or both serve to regulate expression or activation of the actual VDJ recombinase.

Identification and isolation of the RAG genes was based on the knowledge that VDJ recombination activity had only been found in precursor lymphocyte cell lines. This led to a strategy in which a fibroblast-cell line was selected for its ability to inversionally rearrange a VDJ substrate and thereby, express a drug resistant gene.[47] Subsequent transfection approaches led to the cloning of the RAG-1 and RAG-2 genes that, when expressed together, permitted this nonlymphoid cell line to perform VDJ recombination.[45,46] This elegant approach to the isolation of two complementing genes was facilitated by their unique organization: the coding sequence of each is contained within one long exon and the two genes lie, in opposite transcriptional orientation, within several kilobases of each other.[46] As predicted by the distribution of VDJ recombinase activity, the RAG-1 and RAG-2 genes were found to be coexpressed at substantial levels only in primary lymphoid tissues and in cell lines that represent precursor lymphocytes.[22,23] However, expression of one or the other of these genes was found in additional tissues, leading to speculation that one or both of the gene products might have activities in more mature lymphoid cells or in nonlymphoid cells.[48,49]

The RAG genes are conserved in vertebrates but, to date, no close homologs have been found in lower organisms. The RAG-2 gene product has no clear homology to any other gene product.[46] However, the RAG-1 protein does have limited homology to a yeast protein, HPR-1 (high-protein receptor-1), that, in turn, has homology to topoisomerase 1.[50] Furthermore, loss of HPR-1 function in yeast has been shown to increase the rate of homologous recombination.[51] Although homology to HPR-1 has been taken as support for a direct role of RAG-1 in recombination, it is important to point out that even the HPR-1 gene product has not been shown to function directly in a recombination process.

Recent analyses have indicated that the RAG-1 and RAG-2 proteins are expressed predominantly in the cell nucleus, a location consistent with a role either as transcription factors or as VDJ recombinase components.

Despite numerous attempts in several laboratories, neither RAG-1 nor RAG-2 proteins derived from bacterial or mammalian expression systems have been found to exhibit predicted activities, such as sequence-specific DNA binding. Conceivably, such activities will be found as the methods of analysis are modified or improved; it is also possible that these proteins may not function in the absence of higher order structures present in the cell nucleus. Thus, a variety of circumstantial evidence implicates one or both of the RAG gene products as the tissue-specific components of VDJ recombinase,[48] but their precise function has remained difficult to prove.

The acquisition of the ability to recombine transfected VDJ recombination substrates in nonlymphoid cells following introduction of expressed RAG-1 and RAG-2 genes, together with the specific expression patterns of these genes, suggests that the RAG gene products play a central role in initiating the recombination of endogenous VDJ segments.[46] To evaluate this notion unequivocally, and to assess potential nonlymphoid-specific roles for the RAG-1 and RAG-2 gene products, the function of one or the other of these genes was eliminated in mice by embryonic stem cell gene targeting technologies.[52,53] To date, mice lacking either RAG-1 or RAG-2 gene function have identical and very specific phenotypes; both are viable, but show a complete severe combined immune deficiency, due to the apparent inability to initiate the VDJ recombination process in developing T and B cells. Such mice have no mature B or T cells in either primary or peripheral lymphoid tissues and must be maintained in strict barrier facilities to prevent infection. However, tissues from these animals accumulate lymphoid cells that, based on a variety of characteristics, appear to represent very early T- and B-cell progenitors.

Analyses of these primary tissues failed to detect any rearrangements of either endogenous Ig or TCR loci. Furthermore, Abelson murine leukemia virus (A-MuLV) transformants generated from either fetal liver or adult bone marrow of RAG-1 or RAG-2 mutant mice have no rearrangements of any endogenous Ig locus; this is in contrast to those derived from normal mice, which invariably have at least DJ rearrangements. Therefore, in the absence of the RAG-1 or RAG-2 gene products, endogenous (germ-line) Ig (or TCR) loci are inert in developing lymphocytes.[52,53] The specificity of the RAG-2 defect has been demonstrated by transfection of RAG-2 expression vectors into RAG-2/A-MuLV transformants; such cells then acquire the ability to rearrange both transfected VDJ substrates[52] and endogenous J loci efficiently.[53] The latter finding emphasizes that the endogenous Ig loci are fully competent for rearrangement in RAG-2 deficient pre-B cells but can not initiate the process in the absence of the RAG-2 product. Therefore, the severe combined immune deficiency in RAG-1 or RAG-2 deficient mice results from the inability to initiate VDJ rearrangement and, in that regard, is quite distinct mechanistically from the classical murine *scid* mutation (formerly called Swiss-type A gamma globulinemia, a genetic lesion that prevents the normal development of both T and B cells).[54] Because loss of RAG function is not developmentally lethal in mice, it seems likely that some human (autosomal) *scid* mutations might also result from RAG mutations.

Analyses of RAG-1 and RAG-2 deficient mice have, thus far, revealed no abnormalities in any tissue or developmental system outside of the immune system. In particular, the natural killer (NK) and myeloid compartments appear intact in these animals, they are fertile, and there are no obvious neurological defects. The latter finding is particularly significant because RAG-1 was postulated to have a potential role in the development or function of the brain;[48] however, the lack of a detectable phenotype in RAG-1 or RAG-2 deficient mice would appear to eliminate any obvious function for these gene products in the development of the central nervous system. Likewise, these findings question the significance of putative VDJ recombination activity in the brain.[55] However, the possibility of a more subtle function for RAG-1 (or RAG-2) in maintenance of neurological (or other) function,[48] including a role in DNA repair, requires more detailed and long-term analyses of the mutant animals.

Because RAG deficiency is manifested at the earliest lymphocyte precursor stages, current studies of RAG-deficient animals have not eliminated potential roles for these gene products in more mature cells of the immune system. In this regard, a number of B-cell specific processes, including Ig heavy chain class switching and somatic hypermutation (in mammalian B cells) and gene conversion (in chicken B cells), are the most likely candidates to be affected by RAG. Initially, exclusive expression of the RAG-2 gene in the chicken bursa was taken to imply a role for that product in the specifically programmed Ig V gene conversion reaction that takes place in that organ.[49] However, more recent gene targeting studies in chicken bursal lymphoma cell lines have questioned, but not unequivocally eliminated, such a potential function.[56]

All other ideas about potential functions of RAG gene products in such processes are equally speculative. For example, it is notable that most A-MuLV transformed cell lines have both VDJ recombination and class switch activities, suggesting a potential link between these mechanistically distinct B-cell specific recombination processes that could involve RAG-1 or RAG-2.[57] Breeding TCR transgenic constructs into the RAG-2 deficient background fully restores thymic and peripheral T-cell pools with a monoclonal T-cell population. Similar complementation of *scid* mice led to only partial restoration of the primary and peripheral T-cell pools.[58] Such differences may be due to the different nature of the recombination defect prescribed by these two mutations.

NONESSENTIAL TISSUE-SPECIFIC COMPONENTS

The VDJ recombination system employs at least one tissue-specific activity that qualitatively modifies VDJ junctions but is not required for the reaction. The enzyme terminal deoxynucleotidyl transferase (TdT) was proposed to be responsible for the addition of "N" nucleotides at VDJ junctions.[13] Over the years, a large body of circumstantial evidence has further supported this suggestion,[59,60] but unequivocal proof of such a function in the developing immune system probably awaits gene targeting experiments to eliminate TdT function in the animal. Assuming that it is responsible for N-region addition, then differential expression of TdT in particular cell lineages or stages may well underlie the differential appearance of N-regions at the junctions of fetal or adult Ig and TCR repertoires, or in the junctions of Ig heavy and light chains V gene segments. [59-61] There is also potential for activities that result in differential loss of nucleotides in such junctions, although no activity has been as clearly implicated as TdT.

Nontissue-Specific Components

It seems likely that the specific components of VDJ recombinase recruit additional, ubiquitously expressed, cellular activities to perform certain aspects of the process. A spontaneous mouse mutation has provided the first insight into such activities. The murine *scid* mutation was defined as an autosomal recessive mutation that resulted in a general (but often not complete) absence of mature B and T cells due to an impairment in the VDJ recombination process. [54,62] Unlike the RAG mutant pre-B cells, *scid* pre-B cells undergo the initial steps of VDJ recombination relatively efficiently. *Scid* pre-B cells also form RS joins with relatively normal fidelity and efficiency. The *scid* defect is manifested as an inability to form coding joins. [63-66]

Unlike the RAG deficient mice, the severe combined immune deficiency of *scid* mice is "leaky". In other words, *scid* mice do develop populations of peripheral mature lymphocytes, in a time and strain dependent fashion. [67] Although the leakiness of the *scid* mutation may, in some cases, be explained by somatic reversion events, [68] it is probable that much of the leakiness results from the rescue of the liberated coding joins in *scid* prelymphocytes by an illegitimate recombination mechanism that occasionally restores what appear to be normal joins. [69,70] Thus, the lack of leakiness of the RAG mutation compared to the scid mutation can be explained by the nature of the affected activities. The *scid* mutation leads to the generation of free coding ends which, albeit inefficiently, can still be linked to form a "normal" coding join. However, RAG-deficient mice cannot even initiate the VDJ recombination process; therefore, the Ig and TCR variable region loci are as recombinationally inert as any other generic loci in these animals. Such a defect cannot be leaky without reversion of the mutation (which is not possible in the gene-targeted deletions).

The inability of *scid* pre-B cells to form coding joins probably leads to the frequent generation of lethal double strand breaks in the DNA of developing lymphocytes that attempt VDJ recombination. [65] Frequent cell death due to such attempted joining reactions may be one of the reasons that the *scid* defect is difficult to complement with transgenes. [59,71] The homozygous *scid* mutation also has additional manifestations in both lymphoid and nonlymphoid cells, most notably an increased sensitivity to ionizing radiation (for example, an impairment in the ability to repair double strand DNA breaks). [72-74] Thus, it was suggested that the *scid* mutation impairs a more generalized activity involved in double strand break repair, an activity that is recruited by the VDJ recombination system to perform one of the terminal steps in that process.

Mutations in yeast that affect recombination also frequently affect the DNA repair process, particularly the double-strand DNA break repair pathway. [75] VDJ recombination and double strand break repair probably also utilize common enzymatic activities such as exonuclease, polymerase and ligase. To test this idea, a large battery of existing mutant Chinese hamster ovary cell lines [75,76] with known defects in either excision repair (UV sensitivity) or double strand break repair (x-ray sensitivity) were tested for their ability to rearrange induced VDJ recombination substrates following the introduction of RAG expression vectors, and thus to provide the specific VDJ recombination functions of the nonlymphoid cells. [76] None of a variety of different excision repair mutants showed any impairment in the ability to undergo VDJ recombination; however, two of the five double strand break repair mutants tested (Xrs-6 and XR-1) demonstrated a marked decrease in ability to form both coding and RS VDJ joins, while another mutant (V-3) showed a preferential impairment in the joining of coding sequences, reminiscent of the mouse *scid* defect. Each of these lines belongs to a different complementation group,[77] indicating that they are probably encoded by different genes. Given the manifestation of the defect and the evidence from complementation studies, it seems likely that the first two mutations (Xrs-6 and XR-1) affect activities other than the mouse *scid* mutation. Furthermore, revertants of the Xrs-6 and XR-1 mutants obtained by the introduction of specific human chromosomes,[13,36,77] showed a completely normal ability to undergo VDJ recombination when assayed.

The above outlined studies suggest that DNA repair processes and VDJ recombination share a number of components. It is possible that mutated genes that affect DNA repair may exert their effects in direct or indirect fashions, including mutation of an essential component of the reaction (for example, a ligase),[79] a mutation of a factor necessary for expression of a reaction component,[80] or mutation of a factor not involved in the repair process but displaying an activity that interferes with proper expression or activity of a required component. Further definition of activities involved in VDJ recombination may also yield insights into the underlying defects in a number of human diseases that affect the immune system. In this regard, it seems possible that various human diseases that affect both DNA repair processes and lymphocyte development may involve a shared factor.

CONTROL OF VDJ RECOMBINATION

VDJ recombinase activity is controlled in several contexts: the developmental stage (for example, in the assembly of heavy chain variable region genes before those of light chains), lineage (for example, the complete assembly of Ig variable region genes in B cells but not T cells) and allelic exclusion.[35] Since all of these rearrangement events are effected by a common VDJ recombinase, the specificity of its action must be controlled by modulating the accessibility of substrate gene segments.[81] In other words, assuming that VDJ recombinase is expressed constituitively in precursor lymphocytes, then the quality of a particular locus as a substrate determines whether or not it is rearranged.

A paradigm for this concept is provided by comparing the effects of introduced RAG gene expression in VDJ recombinase-negative pre-B cells and nonlymphoid cells. Pre-B-cell lines from RAG-2 deficient mice lack VDJ recombinase activity and display a germ-line configuration at their IgH loci. The generation of VDJ recombination activity in these cells, by the introduction of a RAG-2 expression vector, initiates active rearrangement at the endogenous J_H locus.[82] In contrast, fibroblast cell lines that express VDJ recombination activity through the introduction of RAG-1 and RAG-2 vectors fail to undergo detectable rearrangements of their endogenous Ig loci, despite their ability to rearrange integrated recombination substrates.[83] This difference presumably reflects variations in the accessibility of the J locus in fibroblasts (nonexpressed) and A-MuLV transformants (expressed).

Accessibility Mechanism of VDJ Recombination Control

The susceptibility of V gene segments to undergo efficient rearrangement by VDJ recombinase has been correlated with their transcriptional activity.[35,84] Direct evidence that a transcriptional enhancer can play a role in directing VDJ recombination comes from transgenic mouse studies.[85] These experiments employed a transgene consisting of a TCR-β mini-locus that lacks any known transcriptional enhancer element and that is neither transcribed nor rearranged in any lymphoid or nonlymphoid tissue. However, incorporation into this construct of a segment of DNA that contained the enhancer element from the Ig intron (E*u*) allowed efficient rearrangement and expression of Jβ segments in all developing prelymphocytes. These results were the first unequivocal demonstration that *cis*-acting sequences associated with known transcriptional control elements can target VDJ recombination in normal developing lymphocytes. More recently, other lymphoid-specific enhancer elements, including the TCR Eβ, have also been shown to target rearrangement of this construct in transgenic mice.[82] Furthermore, gene targeting experiments have indicated that the E*u* DNA region plays a similar role in the control of endogenous heavy chain gene assembly; thus, replacement of this DNA region with an expressed Neo[r] gene resulted in a *cis*-acting block of endogenous J$_H$ rearrangement.[82] Together, these findings indicate that the E*u* element influences initiation of J$_H$ rearrangement in the endogenous heavy chain locus; presumably, other enhancer elements play similar roles in the initiation of VDJ rearrangement within other antigen receptor loci.

The exact mechanism by which transcription and/or transcriptional control elements act to promote recombination of VDJ elements remains unclear. A continuing question has been whether the events that confer accessibility upon a locus lead to incidental transcription of that locus, or whether transcription per se confers accessibility for recombination.[84] Temporal uncoupling of transcription and VDJ recombinational accessibility has not been clearly demonstrated. Transcription and homologous recombination have been directly linked in yeast; in this process, transcriptional breakthrough was postulated to promote recombination through alterations in local chromatin structure, including changes in supercoiling of expressed DNA.[86] Unlike VDJ recombination, however, the double strand breaks required to mediate homologous recombination need not be at a precise location (that is, at a heptamer in a recognition sequence). Therefore, the enhancement provided by transcription in this system may simply be a consequence of nonspecific double-strand breaks introduced by components of transcriptional machinery (for example, topoisomerases). Such transcriptionally-induced double-strand breaks may be more relevant to the mechanism of Ig heavy chain class switching, where DNA breaks occur over a region of hundreds of base pairs.

Active transcription has also been correlated with degree of cytosine methylation at CpG residues within a given locus,[87] and recent studies have shown methylation status to have a significant effect on the VDJ recombination potential of substrate gene segments. Expressed loci generally are hypomethylated when compared with silent loci. Hypermethylation of a transgenic substrate occurs via the activity of a strain-specific modifier in certain mouse strains.[88] Recombination of this transgenic substrate occurs in lymphoid tissues, but is restricted primarily to hypomethylated transgene copies. Furthermore, methylation was shown to diminish both VDJ recombinational potential of transiently introduced substrates and their susceptibility to restriction endonuclease digestion within the nucleus.[89] Both effects were more pronounced upon replication of the substrates. These findings suggest that replication of the methylated substrate DNA led to the adoption of less accessible chromatin structure.[89] Differences in nucleosome structures have been reported to exist between hypomethylated CpG islands, which were presumably transcriptionally active, and bulk chromatin;[90] such differences could have implications for accessibility. A protein activity that is capable of binding to methylated DNA has been identified.[91] This activity inhibits transcription from weak promoters, but may be overcome by the addition of an enhancer element that strengthens promoter activity.

The possibility that transcription control of VDJ recombination has further, downstream, roles must also be considered. One possibility is the direct participation of the RNA products of the transcribed loci in VDJ recombination. However, given the assumption that such products should act in *trans*, this notion, in its simplest form, seems to be obviated by the finding that heterozygous disruption of the Eu element in pre-B cells only prevents rearrangement of the targeted allele;[83] nevertheless, a secondary role for this effect, once the locus is rendered accessible, is not inconceivable. Finally, it is clear that protein products derived from complete Ig gene transcripts and, possibly, from germ-line Ig gene transcripts, may transmit signals that regulate VDJ recombination.[61]

Summary

The genes that are necessary and sufficient for generating VDJ recombinase activity in any cell type have been isolated, yet the precise function of their products remains unknown. Clearly, the immediate challenge is to determine whether the RAG gene products represent the tissue-specific components of VDJ recombinase. In that context, another important challenge will be to determine whether VDJ recombination is restricted to certain nuclear locations and, if so, to determine whether such restriction plays any role in the regulation process; for example, by providing a context in which cells can rearrange only one allele at a time.[91] Genetic and biochemical approaches should further define nonspecific components of the reaction; current evidence has already implicated shared components between VDJ recombination and processes such as DNA repair. It seems likely that defects in some such activities may underlie multifaceted diseases that include immunological defects as one component.

References

1. Edelman GM, Cunningham BA, Gail WE, et al. The covalent structure of an entire γ-immunoglobulin molecule. Proc Natl Acad Sci USA 1969; 63: 78-83.
2. Edelman GM, Poulik MD. Studies on structural units of the globulins. J Exp Med 1961; 113: 897-907.
3. Porter RR. The hydrolysis of rabbit γ-globulin and antibodies with crystalline papain. Biochem J 1959; 73: 19-125.

4. Landsteiner K, Chase MW. Experiments on transfer of cutaneous sensitivity to simple compounds. Proc Soc Exp Biol Med 1942; 49: 688-99.

5. Mitchison NA. Passive transfer of transplantation immunity. Nature 1953; 171: 267-70.

6. Gell PG, Benacerraf B. Studies on hypersensitivity. II. Delayed hypersensitivity to denatured proteins in guinea pigs. Immunology 1959; 2: 64-78.

7. Zinkernagel RM, Doherty PC. Immunological surveillance against altered self components by sensitized T lymphocytes in lymphocytic choriomeningitis. Nature 1974; 251: 547-50.

8. Hayday AC, Diamond DJ, Tanigawa G, et al. Unusual organization and diversity of T-cell receptor α chain genes. Nature 1985; 316: 828-35.

9. Winoto A, Mjolsness S, Hood L. Genomic organization of the genes encoding mouse T-cell receptor α chain. Nature 1985; 316: 832-35.

10. Yoshikai Y, Clark SP, Taylor S, et al. Organization and sequence of the variable, joining and constant region genes of the human T-cell receptor α chain. Nature 1985; 316: 837-40.

11. Kronenberg M, Siu G, Hood LE, et al. The molecular genetics of the T-cell antigen receptor and T-cell antigen recognition. Ann Rev Immunol 1986; 4: 529-49.

12. Hedrick SM, Engel I, McElligott DL, et al. Selection of amino acid sequences in the β chain of the T-cell antigen receptor. Science 1988; 39: 1541-44.

13. Alt F, Baltimore D. Joining of immunoglobulin heavy chain gene segments. Implications from a chromosome with evidence of three D-J_H fusions. Proc Natl Acad Sci USA 1982; 79: 4118-22.

14. Gascoigne NR, Chien Y, Becker DM, et al. Genomic organization and sequence of T-cell receptor β chain constant and joining region genes. Nature 1984; 310: 387-89.

15. Malissen M, Minard K, Mjolsness S, et al. Mouse T-cell antigen receptor: Structure and organization of constant and joining gene segments encoding the β polypeptide. Cell 1984; 37: 1101-11.

16. Fink PJ, Matis LA, McElligott DL, et al. Correlation between T-cell specificity and the structure of the antigen receptor. Nature 1986; 321: 219-22.

17. Noonan DJ, Kofler R, Singer PA, et al. Delineation of a defect in T-cell receptor β genes of NZW mice predisposed to autoimmunity. J Exp Med 1986; 163: 644-54.

18. Kotzin BL, Palmer E. The contribution of NZW genes to lupus-like disease in (NZB x NZQ)F_1 mice. J Exp Med 1987; 165: 1237-46.

19. Uematsu Y, Ryser S, Dembic Z, et al. In transgenic mice the introduced functional T-cell receptor β gene prevents expression of endogenous β genes. Cell 1988; 52: 831-40.

20. Chou HS, Nelson CA, Godambe SA, et al. Germline organization of the murine T-cell receptor β chain genes. Science 1987; 238: 545-48.

21. Lai E, Concannon P, Hood L. Conserved organization of the human and murine T-cell receptor β gene families. Nature 1988; 331: 5436-39.

22. Malissen M, McCoy C, Blanc D, et al. Direct evidence for chromosomal inversion during T-cell receptor β-gene rearrangements. Nature 1986; 319: 28-32.

23. Kronenberg M, Goverman L, Haars R, et al. Rearrangement and transcription of the β chain genes of the T-cell antigen receptor in different types of

murine lymphocytes. Nature 1985; 313: 647-50.

24. Okazaki K, Davis DD, Sakano HT. Cell receptor β gene sequences in the circular DNA of thymocyte nuclei: Direct evidence for intramolecular DNA deletion in V-D-J joining. Cell 1987; 49: 477-83.

25. Behlke MA, Henkel TJ, Anderson SJ, et al. Expression of a murine polyclonal T-cell receptor marker correlates with the use of specific members of the Vβ8 gene family subfamily. J Exp Med 1987; 165: 257-63.

26. Kappler JW, Wade T, White J, et al. A T-cell receptor V β segment that imparts reactivity to a class II major histocompatibility complex product. Cell 1987; 49: 263-71.

27. Hayday AC, Saito H, Gillies SD, et al. Structure, organization, and somatic rearrangement of T-cell γ genes. Cell 1985; 40: 259-69.

28. Lefranc MP, Forster A, Rabbitts TH. Genetic polymorphism and exon changes of the constant regions of the human T-cell rearranging gene γ. Proc Natl Acad Sci USA 1986; 83: 9596-9600.

29. Lefranc MP, Forster A, Baer R, et al. Diversity and rearrangement of the human T-cell rearranging γ genes: Nine germ-line variable genes belonging to two subgroups. Cell 1986; 45: 237-44.

30. Huck S, Dariavach P, Lefranc MP. Variable region genes in the human T-cell rearranging γ (TRG) locus: V-J junction and homology with the mouse genes. EMBO J 1988; 7: 719-25.

31. Garman RD, Doherty PJ, Raulet DH. Diversity, rearrangement, and expression of murine T-cell γ genes. Cell 1986; 45: 733-42.

32. Chien YH, Isashima M, Kaplan KB, et al. A new T-cell receptor gene located within the a locus and expressed early in T-cell differentiation. Nature 1987; 327: 677-80.

33. Tonegawa S. Somatic generation of antibody diversity. Nature 1983; 302: 575-82.

34. Lieber MR. Site specific recombination in the immune system. FASEB J 1991; 5: 2934-38.

35. Blackwell TK, Alt FW. Mechanism and developmental program of immunoglobulin gene rearrangement in mammals. Annu Rev Genet 1989; 23: 605-27.

36. Lieber MR, Hesse JE, Mizuuchi K, et al. Lymphoid V(D)J recombination: Nucleotide insertion at signal joints as well as coding joints. Proc Natl Acad Sci USA 1988;85: 8588-92.

37. Hesse JE, Lieber MR, Gellert M, et al. Extrachromosomal DNA substrates in pre-B cells undergo inversion or deletion at immunoglobulin V-(D)-J joining signals. Cell 1987; 49: 775-84.

38. Lafaille JJ, DeCloux A, Bonneville M, et al. Junctional sequences of T-cell receptor γ-delta genes: Implications for γ-delta T-cell lineages and for a novel intermediate of V-(D)-J joining. Cell 1989; 59: 859-65.

39. Akira S, Okazaki K, Sakano H. Two pairs of recombination signals are sufficient to cause immunoglobulin V-(D)-J joining. Science 1987; 238: 1134-37.

40. Hesse JE, Lieber MR, Mizuuchi K, et al. V-(D)-J recombination: A functional definition of the joining signals. Genes Dev 1989; 3: 1053-64.

41. Roth DB, Nakajima PB, Menetski JP, et al. V(D)J recombination in mouse thymocytes: Double-stranded breaks near T-cell receptor delta rearrangement signals. Cell 1992; 69: 41-52.

42. Iwatsato T, Shimizu A, Honjo T, et al. Circular DNA is excised by immunoglobulin class switch recombination. Cell 1990; 62: 143-55.

43. Lewis S, Gellert M. The mechanism of antigen receptor gene assembly. Cell 1989; 59: 585-596.

44. Craig NL. The mechanism of conservative site-specific recombination. Annu Rev Genet 1988; 22: 77-104.

45. Schatz DG, Oettinger MA, Baltimore D. The V(D)J recombination activating gene, RAG-1. Cell 1989; 59: 1035-44.

46. Oettinger MA, Schatz DG, Gorka C, et al. RAG-1 and RAG-2, Adjacent genes that synergistically activate V(D)J recombination. Science 1990; 248: 1517-21.

47. Schatz DG, Baltimore D. Stable expression of immunoglobulin genes V(D)J recombinase activity by gene transfer into 3T3 fibroblasts. Cell 1988; 53: 107-18.

48. Chun JJ, Schatz DG, Oettinger MA, et al. The recombination activating gene-1 (RAG-1) transcript is present in the murine central nervous system. Cell 1991; 64: 189-99.

49. Carlson LM, Oettinger MA, Schatz DG, et al. Selective expression of RAG-2 in chicken B cells undergoing immunoglobulin gene conversion. Cell 1991;64: 201-13.

50. Wang JC, Caron PR, Kim RA. The role of DNA topoisomerases in recombination and genome stability: A double-edged sword? Cell 1990; 62: 403-09.

51. Aguiera A, Klein HL. HPR 1, a novel yeast gene that prevents intrachromosomal excision recombination, shows carboxy-terminal homology to the *Saccharomyces cerevisiae* TOP1 gene. Mol Cell Biol 1990; 10: 1439-46.

52. Shinkai Y, Rathbun G, Lam KP, et al. Rag-2-deficient mice lack mature lymphocytes owing to inability to initiate V(D)J rearrangement. Cell 1992; 68: 855-67.

53. Mombaerts P, Iacomini J, Johnson RS, et al. RAG-1-deficient mice have no mature B and T lymphocytes. Cell 1992; 68: 869-78.

54. Bosma GC, Custer RP, Bosma MJ. A severe combined immunodeficiency mutation in the mouse. Nature 1983; 301: 527-31.

55. Matsuoka M, Nagawa F, Okazaki K, et al. Detection of somatic DNA recombination in the transgenic mouse brain. Science 1991; 254: 81-84.

56. Turka LA, Schatz DG, Oettinger MA, et al. Thymocyte expression of RAG-1 and RAG-2: Termination by T-cell receptor cross linking. Science 1991; 253: 778-81.

57. Lutzker S, Alt FW. In: Berg DE, Howe MM, eds. Mobile DNA. Am Soc Microbiol 1988: 691-714.

58. Scott B, Bluthmann H, Teh HS, et al. The generation of mature T cells requires interaction of the αβ T-cell receptor with major histocompatibility antigens. Nature 1989; 338: 591-94.

59. Blackwell TK, Alt FW. Molecular characterization of the lymphoid V(D)J recombination activity. J Biol Chem 1989; 264: 10327-36.

60. Allison JP, Havran WL. The immunobiology of T cells with invariant γδ antigen receptors. Annu Rev Immunol 1991; 9: 679-703.

61. Rolink A, Melchers F. Molecular and cellular origins of B lymphocyte diversity. Cell 1991; 66: 1081-92.

62. Schuler W, Weiler IJ, Schuler A, et al. Rearrangement of antigen receptor genes is defective in mice with severe combined immune deficiency. Cell 1986; 46: 963-75.

63. Malynn BA, Blackwell TK, Fulop GM, et al. The scid defect affects the final step of the immunoglobulin VDJ recombinase mechanism. Cell 1988; 54: 453-60.

64. Lieber MR, Hesse JE, Lewis S, et al. The defect in murine severe combined immune deficiency: Joining of signal sequences but not coding segments in V(D)J recombination. Cell 1988; 55: 7-18.

65. Blackwell TK, Malynn BA, Pollack RR, et al. Isolation of *scid* pre-B cells that rearrange kappa light chain genes: formation of normal signal and abnormal coding joins. EMBO J 1989; 8: 735-47.

66. Hendrickson EA, Schlissel MS, Weaver DT. Wild-type V(D)J recombination in *scid* pre-B cells. Mol Cell Biol 1990; 10: 5397-5402.

67. Bosma MJ, Carroll AM. The scid mouse mutant: Definition, characterization, and potential uses. Annu Rev Immunol 1991; 9: 323-54.

68. Petrini JHP, Carroll AM, Bosma MJ. T-cell receptor gene rearrangements in functional T-cell clones from severe combined immune deficient (*scid*) mice: Reversion of the scid phenotype in individual lymphocyte progenitors. Proc Natl Acad Sci USA 1990; 87: 3450-55.

69. Ferrier P, Covey LR, Li SC, et al. Normal recombination substrate V_H to DJ_H rearrangements in pre-B-cell lines from *scid* mice. J Exp Med 1990; 171: 1909-21.

70. Bosma GC, Fried M, Custer RP, et al. Evidence of functional lymphocytes in some (leaky) *scid* mice. J Exp Med 1988; 167: 1016-24.

71. Reichman-Fried M, Hardy RR, Bosma MJ. Development of B-lineage cells in the bone marrow of *scid/scid* mice following the introduction of functionally rearranged immunoglobulin transgenes. Proc Natl Acad Sci USA 1990; 87: 2730-34.

72. Fulop GM, Phillips RA. The scid mutation in mice causes a general defect in DNA repair. Nature 1990; 347: 479-82.

73. Biedermann KA, Sun J, Giaccia AJ, et al. *Scid* mutation confers hypersensitivity to ionizing radiation and a deficiency in DNA double-strand break repair. Proc Natl Acad Sci USA 1991; 88: 1394-98.

74. Hendrickson EA, Qin S, Bump EA, et al. A link between double-strand break-related repair and V(D)J recombination: The *scid* mutation. Proc Natl Acad Sci USA 1991; 88: 4061-66.

75. Friedberg EC. Deoxyribonucleic acid repair in the yeast *Saccharomyces cerevisiae*. Microbiol Rev 1988; 52: 70-84.

76. Jeggo PA. Studies on mammalian mutants defective in rejoining double-strand breaks in DNA. Mutat Res 1990; 239: 1-7.

77. Jeggo PA, Tesmer J, Chen DJ. Genetic analysis of ionizing radiation sensitive mutants of cultured mammalian cell lines. Mutat Res 1991; 254: 125-29.

78. Giaccia AJ, Denko N, MacLaren R, et al. Human chromosome 5 complements the DNA double-strand break-repair deficiency and γ-ray sensitivity of the XR-1 hamster variant. Am J Hum Genet 1990; 747: 459-66.

79. Barnes DE, Tomkinson AE, Lehmann AR, et al. Mutations in the DNA ligase I gene of an individual with immunodeficiencies and cellular hypersensitivity to DNA-damaging agents. Cell 1992; 69: 594-605.

80. Jentsch S, McGrath JP, Varshavsky A. The yeast DNA repair gene RAD6 encodes a ubiquitin-conjugating enzyme. Nature 1987; 329: 131-34.

81. Yancopoulos GD, Blackwell TK, Suh H, et al. Introduced T-cell receptor variable gene segments in pre-B cells: Evidence that B and T cells use a common recombinase. Cell 1986; 44: 251-60.

82. Alt FW, Oltz EM, Young F, et al. VDJ recombination. Immunol Today 1992; 13: 306-09.

83. Schatz DG, Oettinger MA, Schlissel MS. V(D)J recombination: Molecular biology and regulation. Annu Rev Immunol 1992; 10: 359-72.

84. Blackwell TK, Moore MW, Yancopoulos GD, et al. Recombination between immunoglobulin variable region gene segments is enhanced by transcription. Nature 1986; 324: 585-87.

85. Ferrier P, Krippl B, Blackwell TK, et al. Separate elements control DJ and VDJ rearrangement in a transgenic recombination substrate. EMBO J 1990; 9: 117-31.

86. Thomas BJ, Rothstein R. Elevated recombination rates in transcriptionally active DNA. Cell 1989; 56: 619-31.

87. Cedar H. DNA methylation and gene activity. Cell 1988; 53: 3-15.

88. Engler P, Haasch D, Pinkert CA, et al. A strain-specific modifier on mouse chromosome 4 controls the methylation of independent transgene loci. Cell 1991; 65: 939-48.

89. Hsieh CC, Lieber MR. CpG methylated minichromosomes become inaccessible for V(D)J recombination after undergoing replication. EMBO J 1992; 11: 315-26.

90. Tazi J, Bird A. Alternative chromatin structure at CpG islands. Cell 1990; 60: 909-919.

91. Boyes J, Bird A. Repression of genes by DNA methylation depends on CpG density and promoter strength: Evidence for involvement of a methyl-CpG binding protein. EMBO J 1992; 11: 327-35.

γδ T Lymphocyte Ontogeny

The γδ T lymphocyte population, a subpopulation of T lymphocytes formed through cell lineages that are independent of the αβ T lymphocyte lineage, consists of multiple subsets with distinct receptor repertoires and homing properties. While the cell sublineage is a critical factor in the determination of homing specificity, both cell sublineage and receptor-dependent selection are instrumental in the determination of the functional repertoire. During thymic ontogeny, rearrangement and cell surface expression of the γ and δ chains precedes that of the α and β chains.[1,2] In peripheral αβ T lymphocytes, some γ genes are often rearranged in a nonproductive, i.e., out-of-frame, form.[3] In contrast, in γδ thymocytes or peripheral γδ T lymphocytes, β genes almost always occur in an incompletely rearranged DJ (D, diversity; J, joining), while α genes are not rearranged. In addition, cells bearing both TCR αβ and γδ or "hybrid" TCRs such as β δ or α γ heterodimers have not been detected in normal animals.[2,4,5] These observations leave little doubt that the αβ and γδ T lymphocyte lineages are segregated from common progenitor cells prior to the expression of either TCR on the cell surface.

What, then, is the critical event that determines cell lineage segregation? Initially, it seemed that γ and δ gene rearrangement was the primary determinant;[2] if the γ and δ gene rearrangements are both productive, then cell-surface expression of γδ TCR occurs, and by analogy with the immunoglobulin system, this inhibits further rearrangement of any other TCR genes. αβ T lymphocytes would thus be generated only from those cells that failed to productively rearrange both γ and δ genes. This model, however, was not supported by transgenic mouse experiments. First, in γδ TCR transgenic mice (KN6 Tg mice) constructed with cosmid clones containing functional rearranged γ and β genes, nearly all γδ T lymphocytes expressed the transgene-encoded γδ TCR and normal numbers of αβ T lymphocytes were present both in the thymus and in the peripheral lymphoid organs of adult mice.[6] These αβ T lymphocytes apparently retained the normal transgenes γ and δ but their RNA transcripts were undetectable. This transcriptional repression of the transgenic γ gene in the αβ T lymphocytes corroborates reports of the silencing of rearranged (both in-frame and out-of-frame) γ genes in the αβT lymphocytes of normal mice,[7] although the $V_2J_2C_2$ γ gene, the protein product of which is rarely expressed on the cell surface, is an exception to this rule.[7] This αβ T lymphocyte specific silencing of Cγ1-associated γ genes is mediated by two DNA elements flanking the enhancer element associated with this gene, and by multiple proteins which interact with these DNA elements.[8]

The function of αβ T lymphocyte specific silencing of γ genes in the segregation of αβ and γδ T lymphocyte lineages was strongly suggested by a second set of γ and δ double transgenic mice in which the downstream silencer element was deleted from the transgene construct.[9] In these transgenic mice, the generation of αβ T lymphocytes was severely retarded, in contrast to the first set of transgenic mice with the complete γ gene-associated silencers. Thus, it has been proposed (figure) that independent of the rearrangement of TCR genes, progenitor cells are split into two lineages: in one the γ silencer machinery remains inactive while in the other it is activated. The γ and δ gene (and perhaps Dβ to Jβ) rearrangements occur in both lineages of cells but only the γ lineage with inactive silencer machinery has the potential to generate γδ T lymphocytes. The surface expression of γδ TCRs prevents, by a feedback mechanism, the completion of β and the initiation of α gene rearrangements, respectively. In the other cell lineage, γδ TCRs will not be expressed on the surface because γ gene expression is blocked at the transcriptional level, and hence the cells may proceed to rearrange Vβ to DJβ and, eventually Vα to Jα; αβ T lymphocytes are generated from this subpopulation upon productive rearrangements of both α and β genes.

It was proposed that a similar silencing element associated with the α gene also affected T lymphocyte development.[10] However, it is unlikely that this silencing element directly affects the segregation of the αβ and γδ T lymphocyte lineages because a gene rearrangement is delayed and, therefore, there is no need to silence the α gene rearrangement at this point of development. It is more likely that the α gene silencer regulates α gene rearrangements relative to β gene rearrangements after the lineage determination is made.[8]

According to another model of αβ T lymphocyte lineage segregation, deletion of the δ locus by a novel recombination determines the commitment of the αβ T lymphocyte lineage.[11] Indeed, there is evidence of deletions in some prothymocytes along the αβ T lymphocyte lineage.[12] However, this model is not compatible with the normal development of αβ T lymphocytes that carry rearranged δ transgenes, therefore, it may be that multiple mechanisms, including both the γ gene silencing and the δ locus deletion, ensure that each lineage expresses only one type of TCR.

γδ T Lymphocyte Subsets

γδ T lymphocytes are not only present in the blood and lymphoid organs such as spleen and lymph nodes but are also disseminated in various tissues, mainly in close association with the epithelial layers that cover the internal and external surface of the body. The γδ cell populations at the various locations represent different γδ cell subsets. They express different TCR repertoires, ranging from monospecific to highly diversified, and differ with regard to their appearance in ontogeny and to thymus dependence. Subset specific surface markers are not yet available and no clear differences have yet been described in functional properties such as cytolytic activity and lymphokine production.

The two γδ cell subsets that appear first in ontogeny are most unusual in that their TCRs show no diversity[13,14] even though they are encoded by rearranged γ and δ genes. One (the Vγ5 subset) is disseminated in the epidermis[13] and the other (the Vγ6 subset) in the mucosal epithelia of the uterus, vagina and tongue.[14] The Vγ5 and the Vγ6 subsets appear in two consecutive waves in the fetal and perinatal thymus, respectively.[15,16] A highly diversified γδ T lymphocyte subset (the Vγ4 subset) is generated later, in the neonatal and adult thymus,[4,17] and exported to the blood and lymphoid organs.[18] This sublineage expresses predominantly Vγ4 and multiple Vδ chains and includes a population of self-reactive cells which express Vγ1 and Vδ6 chains. A fourth γδ cell lineage (the Vγ7 subset is thymus-independent,[19-22] resides mainly in the epithelial layers of the intestine and expresses Lyt2 (CD8a) homodimers[21] and predominantly the Vγ7 chain and Vδ4, Vδ5, Vδ6, and Vδ7 chains which exhibit extensive junctional diversity.[22-25]

The γδ T cells in the liver probably belong to the intestinal lineage since they express CD8 homodimers.[26] However, they preferentially express Vγ1 and Vγ4 rather than Vγ7, which predominates in intestinal γδ T cells. The γδ T cells that have been isolated from the lung[27] and lactating mammary gland[28] express multiple Vγ and Vδ chains and exhibit extensive junctional diversity. At least some γδ T cells in the lung are thymus-independent. It is conceivable that the blood and some organs such as lymph nodes, spleen, lung or mammary gland contain γδ T cells of different sublineages in different proportions.

TCR-Independent Steps in γδ T-cell Subset Development

Do the various γδ T-cell subsets represent distinct sublineages that are derived from different TCR-negative progenitor cells? This is almost certainly true for the intestinal Vγ7 subset, since progenitor cells of this lineage can give rise to mature γδ T cells in the absence of a thymus. Evidence from in vitro and in vivo reconstitution experiments also indicates that the Vγ5 and Vγ6 subsets, generated in the fetal and perinatal thymus, are derived from different progenitor cells than the Vγ4 subset generated in the neonatal thymus. Thus, the progenitors of the adult Vγ4 subset cannot function as progenitors of the fetal Vγ5 subset.[29,30] Adult mice apparently lack both the microenvironment and the progenitor cells required for the generation of the Vγ5 subset.

Does targeting the rearrangement to a specific Vγ gene segment reflect the commitment of a progenitor cell to a particular γδ T-cell subset? Polymerase chain reaction (PCR)-aided Southern blot analysis of the Vγ7 subset colonizing the intestine indicates that this is the case.[25] It has been suggested by limited analysis of nonproductive rearrangements that this may also be true for the progenitor cells of the Vγ4[31-33] and the Vγ5 subsets,[13] although more data are required before a firm conclusion can be drawn. No analogous data are available for the Vγ6 subset. In one study, PCR analysis indicated that there was no good correlation between expression of rearranged Vγ gene segments and their cell-surface expression during the course of fetal thymic development, suggesting that targeted rearrangement is not the primary determinant for the sequential appearance of γδ T-cell subsets.[33] However, interpretation of this type of analysis is complicated by the fact that some of the γ mRNA comes from the progenitors of αβ T cells in which the various Vγ gene segments may not be rearranged according to the same programs that are established in γδ T-cell progenitors. In a recent study, the various rearranged Vγ gene segments in the descendants of 13-day old fetal liver cells that were supplied to the culture of 14-day-old fetal thymuses[8] were measured. It was found that the order of the Vγ rearrangements corresponded to the order of the appearance of the γδ T-cell subsets: the Vγ5 subset appeared first, and the Vγ6 subset second, followed by the Vγ4 subset. These data supported the targeted rearrangement hypothesis.

Homing of the γδ T-cell subsets to and their maintenance in particular peripheral tissues also suggests that differentially targeted rearrangement does occur in the progenitor cells and is part of a coordinated differentiation program that links a specific TCR repertoire to particular functional properties. Bonneville et al[34] demonstrated the TCR-independence of these functional properties for at least two γδ T-cell subsets. They generated TCR-transgenic mice encoding either the TCR of the Vγ5 subset that normally resides in the skin, or the TCR of the Vγ4 subset that normally resides in the blood and lymphoid organs. In these mice, γδ T-cells expressing the "wrong" TCR were found in the intestine and the skin. It is interesting that cells in the intestinal epithelia which expressed the transgenic "skin" TCR did acquire the CD8 marker that is normally expressed by γδ T-cells in the intestine but not expressed by those in the skin.[34] This suggests that the expression of CD8 is not dependent on the specific TCR in the intestinal γδ T-cell subset. However, this is not the case for the two major αβ T-cell subsets, CD4$^+$ and CD8$^+$ cells, whose generation depends on the TCR interaction with MHC class II and class I molecules, respectively.

TCR-Dependent Selection in the Thymus

The fact that the initial step of the γδ sublineage differentiation is TCR-independent does not imply that γδ T-cell sublineage cannot be modified by interactions between maturing T-cells and TCR ligands. Evidence for TCR-mediated thymic selection of γδ T-cells has been obtained by two approaches, one using anti-TCR antibodies to interfere with normal development in vitro and the other relying on mice that express transgenic γδ TCR with specificity for ligands that are expressed by some but not all strains.

The first of these approaches was based on the findings of Asarnow et al[13] and Lafaille et al[35] that the junctional sequences of rearranged Vγ5, Vγ6, and Vδ1 genes in PCR-amplified DNA of fetal thymocytes and epidermal γδ T-cells showed a limitation of junctional diversity in unproductive rearrangements but almost none in productive rearrangements; this suggested that the accumulation of T cells expressing the invariant Vγ5Vδ1 and Vγ6Vδ1 TCRs was due to TCR-mediated positive selection. To prove that this was indeed the case, Itohara and Tonegawa[36] designed an experiment that took advantage of the fact that the two monospecific γδ T-cell subsets can be generated in fetal organ cultures. When they added antibodies against a constant region of the γδ TCR to such cultures they observed an increase in the frequency of productive rearrangements of Vγ5, Vγ6, and Vδ1 junctional sequences. The antibody either mediated positive selection of cells expressing noncanonical TCRs or, more likely, prevented the positive selection of cells expressing canonical TCRs. Whatever the correct explanation might be, the experiment demonstrated that noncanonical TCRs can be generated in the progenitor cells of these two monospecific subsets, i.e., there is a diverse population from which the cells expressing the invariant receptors can be selected. The detection of an increased level of noncanonical, productive Vγ5 to Jγ1 junctional sequences in late fetal liver supports this conclusion.[37]

Since the canonical receptors of these two subsets are identical in the region that corresponds to the third complementarity determining region of the antibody chains, one might speculate that, on the basis of current models of TCR-antigen/MHC protein interactions, that the two $\gamma\delta$ T-cell receptors recognize the same endogenous peptide antigen in the context of different, tissue-specific peptide presenting protein (that is not MHC). The selecting ligands must be expressed in the fetal and perinatal thymus and should be inducible in the epidermis and mucosal epithelia by insults which induce a $\gamma\delta$ T-cell response. Indeed, recent experiments by Allison's group[38] have shown that cells expressing the invariant skin $\gamma\delta$ TCR recognize an endogenous ligand that is inducible in keratinocytes, and that is expressed by fibroblasts treated with tryptic digests of keratinocytes.

Evidence for positive and negative thymic selection of $\gamma\delta$ T cells from the $V\gamma4$ lineage has come from experiments with transgenic mice expressing the rearranged γ and δ genes of the KN6 hybridoma.[39,40] This hybridoma was derived from a C57BL/6 (H-2^b) mouse thymocyte; it expresses α TCR that is typical for the $V\gamma4$ sublineage and recognizes the T27^b gene product, presumably as an autologous peptide-presenting molecule.[41] Interleukin (IL)-2 production is induced in KN6 TCR expressing H-2^d cells when stimulated by spleen cells from H-2^b mice (ligand-positive) but not by spleen cells from H-2^d mice (ligand-negative), which carry a nonfunctional T27 gene. Ligand-positive and ligand-negative TCR transgenic mice had a similar number of thymocytes expressing KN6 TCR but the ligand-negative mice had approximately 10 times fewer spleen cells expressing KN6 TCR.

Pereira et al,[40] by crossing the KN6 TCR transgenic mice with β_2-microglobulin-deficient mice, showed that the development of cells expressing KN6 TCRs depended on positive selection by a protein with β_2-microglobulin-dependent expression. Spleens of β_2-microglobulin-deficient, ligand positive and ligand-negative TCR transgenic mice contained very few cells expressing KN6 TCRs, although large numbers of these cells were found in the thymuses of both types of mice. In an interesting experiment, double staining with a KN6 TCR clonotypic monoclonal antibody (mAb) and mAbs against J11d (a marker for immature thymocytes in the $\alpha\beta$ lineage) showed that the proportion of cells expressing both KN6 TCR and were stained with anti-J11d mAb was about 50% in β_2-microglobulin-positive mice but almost 100% in β_2-microglobulin-negative mice. Hence it was suggested thaT cells expressing KN6 TCR fail to mature in β_2-microglobulin-deficient mice. This finding was further supported by functional studies. Purified $\gamma\delta$ thymocytes from β_2-microglobulin-deficient KN6 TCR transgenic mice failed to proliferate in response to H-2^b spleen cells in the absence of exogenous IL-2 and responded only poorly in the presence of exogenous IL-2. The unresponsive cells from β_2-microglobulin-negative, ligand-negative H-2^d mice resembled the unresponsive cells of the β_2-microglobulin-positive, ligand-positive H-2^b mice but differed from them in that they expressed the transgenic TCR at much higher levels.[40] Essentially the same results were obtained by Wells et al[43] who studied the fate of cells expressing a transgenic TCR with specificity for an undefined T leukemia region product in β_2-microglobulin-positive and β_2-microglobulin-negative mice. Curiously, the TCR transgenes that were used in this study came from a T-cell clone that was derived from nude mice. Therefore one has to assume, that the selection observed by these investigators in the thymus can also take place extrathymically.

As expected from previous studies with αβ TCR transgenic mice[44] the development of CD8$^+$ αβT cells is impaired in β$_2$-microglobulin-deficient mice, which do not express MHC class I proteins.[45] In contrast, no gross abnormalities of γδ T cells were noticed in these mice. This could mean either that most γδ T cells do not depend on selection by a β$_2$-microglobulin-dependent protein or that the majority of γδ T cells depend (as do T cells expressing KN6 TCRs described above) on selection by recognition of β$_2$-microglobulin-dependent proteins. In the latter case then, all γδ T cells in the β$_2$-microglobulin-deficient mice would be derived from β$_2$-microglobulin-unrelated γδ T cells which proliferate to fill up the γδ T-cell compartment. Therefore, the positive selection of Vγ4 sublineage cells, which recognize antigens, resembles the positive selection of αβ T cells, in that cells with highly diversified antigen receptors are selected by the recognition of ligands that are presumably much less diverse. In contrast, positive selection of the monospecific γδ T cells in the fetal thymus is probably mediated by recognition of the same ligands that activate their mature progeny in the periphery.

EXTRATHYMIC TCR-DEPENDENT SELECTION

Differences in the proportion of γδ T cells expressing Vδ4 were observed in the spleens of different mouse strains.[18] In intestinal γδ T-cell populations, expression of the Vδ4 high phenotype was linked to particular MHC class II alleles (dominant in crosses of Vδ4 high and low phenotype), was not dependent on the thymus and was determined by host cells in F1 to parent bone marrow chimeras.[22] In pulmonary γδ T cells from BALB/c but not BALB/b or C57BL/6 mice, two types of TCR sequences referred to as BID and GxYS were repeatedly found.[46-48] These sequences were also found in nude BALB/c but not nude C57BL/6 mice. However, C57BL/6 mice were able to generate both BID and GxYS since BID was found in the fetal C57BL/6 thymus and GxYS in the adult C57BL/6 thymus.[48] In these examples of extrathymic selection it is not clear whether exogenous antigens are involved nor whether immature cells were selected.

HUMAN γδ T CELLS

Human γδ T cells have been extensively studied for their TCR repertoire and putative sublineages. As in mice, rearrangements at the human TCR γ and δ loci also occur in a developmentally ordered fashion.[49] The γδ TCR repertoire that are initially generated in the fetal thymuses of mice and humans is small because rearrangements are targeted to a very limited number of variable gene segments and because junctional diversity is limited. Rearrangements in the thymuses of 8.5- to 15-week-old human embryos involve the joining of Vδ2 to Dδ3 and of Vγ8 or Vγ9 to the Jγ1 cluster.[49] The cells which express these TCR chains may be referred to as the Vγ9Vδ2 subset. There is no evidence for selection of monospecific sublineages in the human thymus. However, from four to six months after birth, rearrangements involve the joining of other Vδ segments, in particular Vδ1 to Dδ1 and Dδ2 and the joining of upstream Vδ gene segments in the Vγ1 family including Vγ2, Vγ3, Vγ5 and Vγ8 to the Jγ2 cluster.[49] The T cells that express these TCR chains may be referred to as the Vγ1Vδ1 subset. The TCR chains of this subset exhibit extensive junctional diversity.

The two major human γδ T-cell subsets Vγ9Vδ2 and Vγ1Vδ2 can be distinguished by monoclonal antibodies such as δTCS1 which recognizes Vδ1Jδ1 and Vδ1Jδ2 but not Vδ1Jδ3, BB3 which recognizes Vδ2, and TiγA which recognizes Vγ9. In the postnatal thymus the Vγ9Vδ2 subset represents about 15% and the Vγ1Vδ1 subset about 80% of all γδ T cells.[50,51] These proportions of thymocytes expressing γδ TCR remain relatively constant throughout adult life. In the blood, however, the Vγ9Vδ2 subset increases with age from approximately 25% in the cord blood to more than 70% in the blood of most adults. There is a corresponding decrease in the Vγ1Vδ1 subset from 50% to less than 30%. Most Vγ9Vδ2 cells become CD45RO⁺ (a probable marker for memory cells), while most Vγ1Vδ1 subset T cells remain CD45RO⁻. The accumulation of CD45RO⁺ (naive cells) Vγ9Vδ2 cells in the blood is thought to be the result of stimulation of mature cells by common ligands for Vγ9Vδ2 TCRs, such as the superantigen staphylococcal enterotoxin-A[52] and unidentified components of mycobacteria,[53,54] *Plasmodium falciparum*[55] or cell lines such as Molt4[53] and Daudi,[56,57] which may express superantigens. Selection of the predominant Vδ T-cell subset in adult human blood by superantigens is consistent with the extensive junctional diversity of their TCRs. Expansion of antigen-specific γδ T-cell clones has also been reported. For example, γδ T-cell subsets with limited diversity can be a striking observation in patients with sarcoidosis.[58] Sequencing of mRNA obtained from the blood of two patients revealed identical junctions in 84% and 54% of Vγ9 transcripts. In one case, 67% of Vγ9 transcripts from bronchoalveolar lavage showed the same junctional sequence and this was identical to the predominant sequence in the blood.

REFERENCES

1. Raulet DH, Garman RD, Saito HY, et al. Developmental regulation of T-cell receptor gene expression. Nature 1985; 314: 103-07.

2. Pardoll DM, Fowlkes BJ, Bluestone JA, et al. Differential expression of two distinct T-cell receptors during thymocyte development. Nature 1987; 326: 79-81.

3. Heilig JS, Tonegawa S. T-cell γ gene is allelically but not isotypically excluded and is not required in known functional T-cell subsets. Proc Natl Acad Sci USA 1987; 84: 8070-74.

4. Itohara S, Nakanishi N, Kanagawa O, et al. Monoclonal antibodies specific to native murine T-cell receptor γδ: Analysis of γδ T-cells in thymic ontogeny and peripheral lymphoid organs. Proc Natl Acad Sci USA 1989; 86: 5094-98.

5. Hochstenbach F, Brenner MB. T-cell receptor δ chain can substitute for α to form a βδ heterodimer. Nature 1989; 340: 562-65.

6. Ishida I, Verbeck S, Bonneville M, et al. T-cell receptor γδ and γ transgenic mice suggest a role of a γ gene silencer in the generation of αβ T-cells. Proc Natl Acad Sci USA 1990; 87: 3067-71.

7. Heilig JS, Tonegawa S. Diversity of murine γ genes and expression in fetal and adult T lymphocytes. Nature 1986; 322: 836-40.

8. Hass W, Tonegawa S. Development and selection of γδ T cells. Cur Opin Immunol 1992; 4: 147-55.

9. Bonneville M, Ishida I, Mombaerts P, et al. Blockade of αβ T-cell development by TCR γδ transgenes. Nature 1989; 342: 931-32.

10. Winoto A, Baltimore D. αβ lineage-specific expression of the γ T-cell receptor gene by nearby silencers. Cell 1989; 59: 649-55.

11. De Villartay JP, Cohen DL. Gene regulation within the TCR-γδ locus by specific deletion of the TCR-δ cluster. Res Immunol 1990; 141: 618-23.

12. De Villartay JP, Mossalayi D, deChasseval R, et al. The differentiation of human prothymocytes along the TCR-αβ pathway in vitro is accompanied by the site-specific deletion of the TCR-δ locus. Int Immunol 1991; 3: 1301-05.

13. Asarnow DM, Kuziel WA, Bonyhadi M, et al. Limited diversity of γδ antigen receptor genes of Thy-1[+] dendritic epidermal cells. Cell 1988; 55: 837-47.

14. Itohara S, Farry AG, Lafaille JJ, et al. Homing of a γδ thymocyte subset with homogenous T-cell receptors to mucosal epithelial. Nature 1990; 343: 754-57.

15. Harvan WL, Allison JP. Developmentally ordered appearance of thymocytes expressing T-cell antigen receptors. Nature 1988; 335: 443-45.

16. Ito K, Bonneville M, Takagaki Y, et al. Different γδ T-cell receptors are expressed on thymocytes at different stages of development. Proc Natl Acad Sci USA 1989; 86: 631-35.

17. Takagaki Y, Nakanishi N, Ishida I, et al. T-cell receptor [+]γ and [-]δ genes preferentially utilized by adult thymocytes for the surface expression. J Immunol 1989; 142: 2212-21.

18. Bluestone JA, Cron RQ, Barrett TA, et al. Repertoire development and ligand specificity of murine TCR γδ cells. Immunol Rev 1991; 120: 5-33.

19. Bandeira, Itohara S, Bonneville M, et al. Extrathymic origin of intestinal intraepithelial lymphocytes bearing T-cell antigen receptor γδ. Proc Natl Acad Sci USA 1991; 88: 43-47.

20. Mosley RL, Styre D, Klein JR. Differentiation and functional maturation of bone marrow-derived intestinal epithelial T-cells expressing membrane T-cell receptor in athymic radiation chimeras. J Immunol 1990; 145: 1369-75.

21. Guy-Grand D, Malassis-Seris M, Briottet C, et al. Cytotoxic differentiation of mouse gut thymodependent and independent intraepithelial T lymphocytes is induced locally. Correlation between functional assays, presence of perforin and granzyme transcripts and cytoplasmic granules. J Exp Med 1991; 173: 1549-52.

22. Lefrancois L, Lecorre R, Mayo J, et al. Extrathymic selection of TCR γδ[+] cells by class II major histocompatibility complex molecules. Cell 1990; 63: 333-40.

23. Bonneville M, Janeway CA Jr, Ito K, et al. Intestinal intraepithelial lymphocytes are a distinct set of γδ T-cells. Nature 1988; 336: 479-81.

24. Kyes S, Carfew E, Carding SR, et al. Diversity in T-cell receptor γ gene usage in intestinal epithelium. Proc Natl Acad Sci USA 1989; 86: 5527-31.

25. Takagaki Y, Decloux A, Bonneville M, et al. Diversity of γδ T-cell receptors on murine intestinal intraepithelial lymphocytes. Nature 1989; 339: 712-14.

26. Ohteki T, Abo T, Seki S, et al. Predominant appearance of γδ T lymphocytes in the liver of mice after birth. Eur J Immunol 1991; 21: 1733-40.

27. Augustin A, Kuno RT, Sim GK. Resident pulmonary lymphocytes expressing the γδ T-cell receptor. Nature 1989; 340: 239-41.

28. Reardon C, Lefrancois L, Farr A, et al. Expression of γδ T-cell receptors on lymphocytes from the lactating mammary gland. J Exp Med 1990; 172: 1263-66.

29. Havran WL, Allison JP. Origin of Thy-1$^+$ dendritic epidermal cells of adult mice from fetal thymic precursors. Nature 1990; 344: 68-70.

30. Ikuta K, Kina T, MacNeil I, et al. A developmental switch in thymic lymphocyte maturation potential occurs at the level of hematopoietic stem cells. Cell 1990; 62: 863-74.

31. Kranz DM, Saito H, Heller M, et al. Limited diversion of the rearranged T-cell γ gene. Nature 1985; 313: 752-55.

32. Korman AJ, Marusic-Galesic S, Spencer D, et al. Predominant variable region gene usage by γδ T-cell receptor-bearing cells in the adult thymus. J Exp Med 1988; 168: 1021-40.

33. Carding SR, Kyes S, Jenkinson EJ, et al. Developmentally regulated fetal thymic and extrathymic T-cell receptor γδ gene expression. Gene Dev 1990; 4: 1304-15.

34. Bonneville M, Itohara S, Krecko EG, et al. Transgenic mice demonstrate that epithelial homing of γδ T cells is determined by cell lineages independent of T-cell receptor specificity. J Exp Med 1990; 171: 1015-26.

35. Lafaille JL, Decloux A, Bonneville M, et al. Junctional sequences of T-cell receptor γδ genes: implications for γδ T-cell lineages and for a novel intermediate of V-(D)-J joining. Cell 1989; 59: 857-70.

36. Itohara S, Tonegawa S. Selection of γδ T cells with canonical T-cell antigen receptors in fetal thymus. Proc Natl Acad Sci USA 1990; 87: 7935-38.

37. Kyes S, Pao W, Hayday A. Influence of site expression on the fetal γδ T-cell receptor repertoire. Proc Natl Acad Sci USA 1991; 88: 7830-33.

38. Havran WL, Chien YH, Allison JP. Recognition of self antigens by skin-derived T cells with invariant γδ antigen receptors. Science 1991; 252: 1430-32.

39. Bonneville M, Ishida I, Itohara S, et al. Self-tolerance to transgenic γδ T cells by intrathymic inactivation. Nature 1990; 344: 163-65.

40. Pereira P, Zijlstra M, McMaster J, et al. Blockade of transgenic γδ T-cell development in β$_2$-microglobulin deficient mice. EMBO J 1992; 11: 25-31.

41. Ito K, Van Kaer L, Bonneville M, et al. Recognition of the product of a novel MHC TL region gene (27^b) by a mouse γδ T-cell receptor. Cell 1990; 62: 549-56.

42. Dent AL, Matis LA, Hooshmand F, et al. Self-reactive γδ T cells are eliminated in the thymus. Nature 1990; 343: 714-19.

43. Wells FB, Gahm SJ, Hedrick SM, et al. Requirement for positive selection of γδ receptor bearing T cells. Science 1991; 253: 903-05.

44. Von Boehmer H. Development biology of T cells in T-cell receptor transgenic mice. Annu Rev Immunol 1990; 8: 531-56.

45. Zijlstra M, Bix M, Simister NE, et al. β$_2$-microglobulin deficient mice lack CD4⁻8$^+$ cytolytic T cells. Nature 1990; 344: 742-46.

46. Sim GK, Augustin A. Dominantly inherited expression of BID, an invariant undiversified T-cell receptor δ chain. Cell 1990; 61: 397-405.

47. Sim GK, Augustin A. Dominant expression of the T-cell receptor BALB invariant δ (BID) chain in resident pulmonary lymphocytes is due to selection. Eur J Immunol 1991; 21: 859-61.

48. Sim GK, Augustin A. Extrathymic positive selection of γδ T cells. J Immunol 1991; 146: 2439-45.

49. Krangel MS, Yssel H, Brocklehurst C, et al. A distinct wave of human T-cell receptor γδ lymphocytes in the early fetal thymus: evidence for controlled gene rearrangements and cytokine production. J Exp Med 1990; 172: 847-59.

50. Porcelli S, Brenner B, Band H. Biology of the human γδ T-cell receptor. Immunol Rev 19γ1; 120: 137-83.

51. Casorati G, Delibero G, Lanzavecchia A, et al. Molecular analysis of human γδ clones from the thymus and peripheral blood. J Exp Med 1989; 170: 1521-35.

52. Rust CJJ, Verreck F, Victor H, et al. Specific recognition of staphylococcal enterotoxin A by human T cells bearing receptors with the Vγ9 region. Nature 1990; 346: 572-74.

53. De Libero G, Casorati G, Giachino C, et al. Selection by two powerful antigens may account for the presence of the major population of human peripheral γδ T cells. J Exp Med 1991; 173: 1311-22.

54. Kabelitz D, Bender A, Prospero T, et al. The primary response of human γδ⁺ T cells to Mycobacterium tuberculosis is restricted to Vγ9-bearing cells. J Exp Med 1991; 173: 1331-38.

55. Goerlich R, Hacker G, Pfeffer K, et al. Plasmodium falciparum merozites primarily stimulate the Vγ9 subset of human γδ T cells. Eur J Immunol 1991; 21: 2613-16.

56. Strum E, Braakman E, Fisch P, et al. Human Vγ9 Vδ2 T-cell receptor-γδ lymphocytes show specificity to Daudi Burkitt's lymphoma cells. J Immunol 1990; 145: 3202-08.

57. Fisch P, Malkovsky M, Braakman E, et al. γδ T-cell clones and natural killer cell clones mediate distinct patterns of nonmajor histocompatibility complex-restricted cytolysis. J Exp Med 1990; 171: 1567-79.

58. Tamura N, Holroyd KJ, Banks T, et al. Diversity in junctional sequences associated with the common human Vγ9 and Vδ2 gene segments in normal blood and lung compared with the limited diversity in a granulomatous disease. J Exp Med 1990; 172: 169-181.

CHAPTER 11

SURGICAL THYMECTOMY AND THE IMMUNE RESPONSE

The first hints that the thymus might in some way be involved in protecting the individual against disease was first seen in the early 1800s works of Lucae[1] and Rush.[2] Later, His[3,4] clearly saw the relationship between the thymus and lymph nodes, tonsils, spleen and Peyer's patches, with all having similar cell types. The connection between the various types of leukemia and their pathological characteristics with an abnormal thymus were initially noted by Virchow,[5] Wilks[6] and Paltauf.[7] In the early 20th century, a number of researchers noted that removal of the thymus in early life not only led to a cachectic condition,[8,9] but also impaired resistance to disease. Cozzolino[10] observed that thymectomized rabbits have a decreased resistance to diphtheria toxin. As early as 1909, Soli[11] maintained that the thymus was important for protection against infection, proper bone development, and sexual maturation. Interestingly, Caridroit observed in his studies that deficiency diseases were more severe in thymectomized animals.[12] Klose and Vogt[13] noted that their cachectic dogs were subject to many pathogenic infections before eventually succumbing.

In 1911, Rohdenberg et al[14] found that thymectomized rats were more receptive to tumor transplants, while removing other glands, such as the testes, seemed to enhance resistance to cancer. These studies encouraged Rohdenberg and his colleagues to provide thymus glands as an oral therapy to some 48 human carcinoma patients, with some slight temporary slowing of the tumor growth. A year later, Magnini[15,16] reported that a simple thymic extract given to thymectomized rats not only prevented wasting disease but also increased resistance to a transplanted carcinoma. Maeda[17] confirmed this work as well as that of Rohdenberg et al.[14] In 1930, Babes[18] also observed that the lack of a thymus gland led to a decrease in resistance to tumor implantation. Parhon proposed in 1937 that the thymus had an antineoplastic function.[19] Over the period from 1910 to 1940, there was a general recognition that the thymus was somehow involved in the body's defense against disease, although the nature of this gland as a key element in the immune system was not recognized.[11]

It has been recognized for some time that foreign protein, be it an allograft, pathogen, foreign protein, or tumor cell, invokes a reaction from the lymphocytes and lymphoid tissue,[20,21] and that these immune responses[22] are characterized by specificity.[23] In 1925, Goldner noted that there are different populations of lymphocytes with some types being more resistant to accidental involution of the thymus than others.[24] Emmel et al[25] simultaneously observed that leukocytes migrated to those areas of the body where a functional need arises. Injections of antigens would also lead to a proliferation of lymphoid cells[26] and enhanced phagocytosis.[27]

As awareness grew that the antibody-antigen reaction is fundamental to an immune response and that the thymus plays an important role in immune defenses, studies were undertaken to characterize their interrelationships. A number of investigators found that the thymus gland generally does not respond to antigenic stimulation[28,29] and does not normally produce antibodies.[30,31] However, the direct injection of antigens into the thymus itself stimulates the development of germinal centers and antibody formation.[29,32]

It is thus generally concluded that a barrier to antigen exists between the circulatory system and the thymic parenchyma.[29,33] In 1961, Fichtelius et al[34] published a seminal paper noting that even though the spleen is the major site of circulating antibody,[35,36] the thymus plays a role in antibody formation, since thymectomy dramatically reduces the amount detected. When used at the proper dosage, the drug colchicine was found to lyse lymphocytes in the thymus and other lymphoid organs. Colchicine-treated rats dramatically lost thymus weight due to lymphocyte destruction, without an increase in antibody levels.[37] This indicated that the lymphocytes were not releasing antibody when lysed.

The 1960s witnessed a tremendous surge in the study of the relationship of the thymus to the immune response. It was established that defects in the immune system are instrumental in the initiation of infectious and malignant diseases.[38-43] It also became recognized that the rodent fetal-neonatal thymus initially lacks immunocompetence but matures over a period of time after birth.[44-50] For instance, inoculation of a mouse embryo with tumor cells leads to an acquired tolerance toward that type of tumor; that is, later injection of tumor cells does not trigger a normal immune response.[45,46] Similarly, inoculation of neonates with protein antigens abrogates a response to a later injection of the same substance.[47-51] In 1957, Dixon et al[52] showed that it was possible to transfer an immune reaction with lymphoid cells from a sensitized to a nonsensitized animal. Thymic lymphocytes were demonstrated to act slower than peripheral lymphocytes in initiating an immune response, thus indicating a degree of immaturity in the former.[53] In 1959, Billingham and Brent offered convincing proof that some, but not all of the thymic lymphocytes are immunologically competent.[54]

One method of determining the essential nature of the thymus was to remove it, and then measure changes in the immune function using a repertory of test methods developed in the late 1950s and early 1960s. It should be noted that different species show varying degrees of immune competence at birth. Most rodent thymuses are relatively immature, while the rabbit, sheep, and human show a considerably greater immune response at birth such that thymectomy at some time in early life no longer leads to immune incompetence but only varying degrees of immune deficiency, inversely proportional to age. Therefore, Table 1 should be considered a rather general, but not absolute, overview of the effect of thymectomy in other species besides the mouse.

Relationship of the Thymus to Oncogenesis

Although the function of the thymus in the host's immunologic interaction with a tumor remains obscure, ample experimental and clinical evidence indicates that both the presence of thymic abnormalities and the removal of the thymus have crucial roles in the development of extrathymic tumors. In diseases with an increased risk of neoplasia, thymic pathology is often present and conversely following experimental thymectomy, there is a marked alteration in the growth of neoplasms. Of considerable interest, because of the potential for clinical application, are the reports indicating that thymectomy may have an inhibitory effect on the development of certain neoplasms.

Through its control of T cells and their immunological mechanisms, the thymus is considered to inhibit neoplastic growth (the concept of immunological surveillance[81]). Indeed, reports indicate that increased tumor growth can occur after thymectomy.[82] However, although tumor-specific cytolytic activity by T cells has been demonstrated in in vitro studies, in vivo studies show that, contrary to expectations, tumor growth is frequently inhibited in thymectomized animals. Experimental thymectomy was followed by an alteration in the incidence of tumors and a reduced occurrence of mammary tumors, lymphomas and leukemias.[83-85] It appears, therefore, that according to conditions, the thymus may have both an enhancing and an inhibiting effect on neoplastic growth. Since naturally occurring tumors express either weak or no cell-surface neoantigens, thymus-dependent rec-

---

Table 1. Effect of neonatal thymectomy on immune response of the mouse

Function	Effect	Reference
Viral transformation	Enhanced	55-58
Thyroid gland	Atrophication	59
Secondary sex characteristics	Lack of development	59
Plasma cell formation	Little or no change	60,61
Immunoglobulins	No change or completely absent, depending on animal species and immunoglobulin type	62-65
Lymphocyte production	Severe decrease	8,9,66-71
Lymph node weight	Reduced	68
Primary response to antigen	Reduced	62-64,72-74
Heterograft rejection	Impaired	75-78
Resistance to infectious disease, including those arising from usually nonpathogenic viruses	Lowered	79,80

ognition of neoplastic mutant cells may not occur, and thus the thymus may not inhibit tumor growth. Persistent thymic abnormalities and the presence of a thymoma have also been linked to an increased susceptibility to neoplasia.[86] The consistent observations indicating that thymectomy protect against neoplasms in some animal models support the suggestion[87] that thymic suppressor cells inhibit the activity of tumor-cytotoxic cells, and that thymectomy, by abolishing suppression, protects against neoplasia.

Olsson et al[88] pointed out that thymus-deprived lymphocyte cells have a cytolytic potential against malignant cells with surface tumor neoantigens. Thymectomy permitted the inhibition of leukemia growth to be mediated apparently by cytotoxic lymphoid cells in AKR mice. It was noted that thymectomy could also adversely result in autoimmune reactions. However, the experience with thymectomy in patients with myasthenia gravis has not been followed by an increased incidence of autoimmune phenomena. Indeed, thymectomy seems to protect against other autoimmune diseases.[89]

Subsequent reports have also shown a protective effect of thymectomy for other than mammary tumors, lymphomas and leukemias.[83] Reinisch et al[87] reported that thymectomy in young adult life prevents subsequent development of murine sarcomas. In their study, 25 of 30 sham thymectomized mice given murine sarcoma virus developed lymphoma by 10 months of age, but only 4 of the 30 mice that had also undergone thymectomy developed tumors. They suggested that thymectomy either removed suppressor cells with a resulting enhanced cytolytic T-cell activity against syngeneic tumor cells, or removed a lymphoid organ known to be a site of viral replication (thymus). This concept is supported by the demonstration that adult thymectomy decreases suppressor T-cell activity in adult animals while increasing helper cells and cytolytic T-cell activity.[90]

Experimental thymectomy in breast cancer also appears to not only decrease the risk of development of breast cancer but appears to affect the course of the disease following tumor appearance. Both neonatal and adult thymectomy have most consistently inhibited growth of mammary neoplasms even after the tumor has developed.[91] Prolongation of survival in C3H MTV+ mice following thymectomy and tumor removal suggests that thymectomy may have an adjuvant role with surgical ablation of the tumors.[91] Thymectomy also decreases the incidence and delays the appearance of spontaneous, virus-induced, chemically induced, and transplantable mammary tumors.[84,85] Roubinian et al[92] suggested that mammary tumorigenesis especially may be influenced by a balance of thymic regulatory factors.

While the effects of thymectomy in experimental oncogenesis have been extensively investigated,[82-84] there is a remarkable paucity of such reports in relation to human tumors. However, it appears that the presence of thymic pathology is associated with an increased frequency of extrathymic neoplasms and that thymectomy is not associated with an increased risk of oncogenesis.[93,94] In fact, as for experimental tumors,[95] it appears that thymectomy may play a protective role. This concept is supported by the inhibition of neoplastic growth following thymectomy in myasthenic patients. The incidence of associated neoplasms was less frequent in 2,136 myasthenic patients followed at Mount Sinai Medical Center following thymectomy than in those not receiving thymectomy, regardless of age.[96]

IMPLICATIONS

Most of the reports on thymectomy in oncogenesis deal with the protective effect of thymectomy against subsequent development of tumors. However, thymectomy may have a protective effect against neoplasia even after the development of an extrathymic neoplasm, since Peer et al[91] reported that thymectomy combined with tumor excision in C3H mice with mammary tumors resulted in prolonged absolute survival, disease-free survival, and survival following recurrence of the tumor. Results in human patients have been very limited. Goldstein and Mackay[100] suggested that thymectomy should be performed before the onset of lymphosarcoma and chronic lymphocyte leukemia. Patey[98] reported a benign clinical course in patients with Hodgkin's disease who underwent thymectomy.

Since thymectomy results in the earlier remission of symptoms of myasthenia gravis in a greater proportion of patients,[96] and inhibits the development of extrathymic malignant neoplasms, early thymectomy should be a treatment of choice before there is further progression of disease. There are reports that thymectomy also arrests the development of symptoms of other autoimmune diseases. Good results have been achieved with thymectomy in Behcet's disease, ulcerative colitis, chronic thyroiditis, systemic lupus erythematosus, autoimmune hemolytic anemia, and Sjogren's syndrome.[89] In most of these autoimmune syndromes there is also a high incidence of associated extrathymic neoplasms.[101]

REFERENCES

1. Lucae SC. Anatomische Bemerkungen uber die Hohlen der Thymus. Erlangen Abh 1812; 2: 22-24.
2. Rush B. An Inquiry into the use of the thymus gland. Med Rep NY 1811; 2: 83-85.
3. His W. Beitrage zur Kenntniss der zum Lymphsystem gehorigen Drusen. Z Wiss Zool 1860; 10: 333-36.
4. His W. Beitrage zur Kenntniss der zum Lymphsystem gehorigen Drusen. 3. Ueber den Bau der lymphdrusen. Z Wiss Zool 1861; 11: 65-68.
5. Virchow R. Ueber bewegliche thierische Zellen. Arch Pathol Anat Physiol (Virchows) 1863; 28: 237-41.
6. Wilks S. Enlargement of the lymphatic glands and spleen. Guy's Hosp Rep 1865; 11: 56-59.
7. Paltauf A. Ueber die Bezeihungen der Thymus zum plotzlichen Tod. Wien Klin Wochenschr 1890; 9: 172-76.
8. Roosa RA, Wilson D, Defendi V. Effect of neonatal thymectomy in hamsters. Fed Proc Ped Am Soc Exp Biol 1963; 22: 599-605.
9. Defendi V, Roosa RA, Koprowski H. Effect of thymectomy at birth on response to tissue, cells and virus antigens. In: Good RA, Gabrielsen AE, eds. The Thymus in Immunobiology. New York: Harper & Row, 1964: 504-34.
10. Cozzolino O. Intorno agli effetti dell'estirpazione del timo nei giovani conigli. Pediatria 1903; 2: 144-53.
11. Soli V. Contribution a la connaissance de la fonction du thymus chez le poulet et chez quelques mammiferes. Arch Ital Biol 1909; 52: 353-55.
12. Caridroit F. Effects de la thymectomie su le rat alimente au riz pali. Cr Soc Biol 1924; 90: 1330-34.
13. Klose H, Vogt H. Klinik und Biologie der Thymusdruse besonderer

Berucksichtigung, ihrer Beziehungen zu Knochen und Nervensystem. Beitr Klin Chir. 1910; 69: 1-6.

14. Rohdenberg GL, Bullock FD, Johnston PJ. The effects of certain internal secretions on malignant tumors. Arch Int Med 1911; 4: 491-98.

15. Magnini M. Le funzioni del timo ed i rapporti fra timo e milza. Arch Fisiol 1912; 11: 333-37.

16. Magnini M. Development of neoplasms in thymectomized rats. Tumori 1913; 2: 325-26.

17. Maeda K. Relation between thymus gland and growth of tumor. Trans Jpn Pathol Soc 1930; 20: 659-61.

18. Babes A. Thymus et cancer du gordron. CR Soc Biol 1930; 103: 165-69.

19. Parhon CI. Apercu general sur le thymus au point de vue endocrinologique. Bull Men Soc Endocrinol 1937; 7: 181-85.

20. Wiseman BK. The induction of lymphocytosis and lymphatic hyperplasia by means of parentally administered protein. J Exp Med 1931; 53: 499-508.

21. Rich AR, Lewis MR, Wintrobe MM. The activity of the lymphocyte in the body's reaction to foreign protein, as established by the identification of the acute splenic tumor cell. Bull Johns Hopkins Hosp 1939; 65: 311-17.

22. Medawar PB. The behavior and fate of skin autografts and skin homografts in rabbits. J Anat 1944; 78: 176-87.

23. Furth J, Kabat EA. Immunolgical specificity of material sedimentable at high speeds present in normal and tumor tissue. J Exp Med 1941; 74: 247-56.

24. Goldner J. Reaktionen der thymus wahrend der Knochenbruche. Arch Mikrosk Anat 1925; 104: 72-75.

25. Emmel VE, Weatherford HL, Streicher MH. Leukocytes and lactation. Am J Anat 1926;38: 1-16.

26. Fichtelius KE, Hassler O. Influence of pertussis vaccine on the lymphocyte production in adrenalectomized rats. Acta Pathol Microbiol Scand 1958; 42: 189-92.

27. Bailiff RN. Reaction patterns of the reticuloendothelial system under stimulation. Ann NY Acad Sci 1960; 88: 3-12.

28. Marshall AHE, White RG. The immunological reactivity of the thymus. Br J Exp Pathol 1961; 42: 379-84.

29. Sainte-Marie G. Antigen penetration into the thymus. J Immunol 1963; 9: 840-48.

30. Thorbecke GJ, Keuning FJ. Antibody formation in vitro by hematopoietic organs after subcutaneous and intravenous immunization. J Immunol 1953; 70: 129-37.

31. Harris TN, Rhodes J, Stokes J. A study of the role of thymus and spleen in the formation of antibodies in the rabbit. J Immunol 1948; 58: 27-39.

32. Stoner RD, Hale WM. Antibody production by the thymus and Peyer's patches to intraocular transplants. J Immunol 1955; 75: 203-09.

33. Raviola E, Karnovsky MJ. Evidence for a blood thymus barrier using electron-opaque tracers. J Exp Med 1972; 136: 466-75.

34. Fichtelius KE, Laurell G, Phillipson L. The influence of thymectomy on antibody formation. Acta Pathol Microbiol Scand 1961; 51: 81-84.

35. Winebright J, Fitch FW. Antibody formation in the rat. I. Agglutinin response to particulate flagella from Salmonella typhosa. J Immunol 1962; 89: 891-96.

36. Fagraeus A. The plasma cellular reaction and its reaction to the formation of

antibodies in vitro. J Immnuol 1948; 58: 1-8.

37. Fagraeus A, Gormsen H. The effect of colchicine on circulating antibodies, antibody producing tissues and blood cells in the rat. Acta Pathol Microbiol Scand 1953; 33: 421-24.

38. Chediak M. Nouvelle anomalie leucocytaire de caractere constitutionnel et familial. Rev Haematol 1952; 7: 362-65.

39. Good RA, Zak SJ. Disturbances in gammaglobulin synthesis as "experiments of nature". Pediat J 1956; 18: 109-18.

40. Gitlin D, Vawter G, Craig JM. Thymic alymphoplasia and congenital aleukocytosis. Pediatrics 1964; 184: 1964-69.

41. Law LW. Studies of thymic function with emphasis on the role of the thymus in oncogensis. Cancer Res 1966; 26: 551-59.

42. Osoba D. The function of the thymus. Can Med Assoc J 1966; 94: 488-93.

43. Miller JFAP. The thymus, yesterday, today, and tomorrow. Lancet 1967; 2: 1299-1303.

44. Archer OK, Pierce JC. Role of thymus in development of immune response. Fed Proc Fed Am Soc Exp Biol 1961; 20: 26-32.

45. Koprowski H. Actively acquired tolerance to a mouse tumor. Nature 1955; 175: 1087-89.

46. Aust JB, Martinez C, Bittner JJ, et al. Tolerance in pure strain newborn mice to tumor homografts. Proc Soc Exp Biol Med 1956; 92: 27-31.

47. Pietra G, Spencer K, Shubik P. Response of newly born mice to a chemical carcinogen. Nature 1959; 183: 1689-92.

48. Dixon FJ, Maurer PH. Immunologic unresponsiveness in rabbits produced by neonatal injections of defined antigens. J Exp Med 1955; 108: 227-34.

49. Bortin MM, Rimm AA, Saltzstein EC. Ontogenesis of immune capability of murine bone marrow cells and spleen cells against transplantation antigens. J Immunol 1969; 103: 683-89.

50. Boraker DK, Hildemann WH. Maturation of alloimmune responsiveness in mice. Transplantation 1965; 3: 202-07.

51. Smith RT, Bridges RA. Immunological unresponsiveness in rabbits produced by neonatal injections of defined antigens. J Exp Med 1958; 108: 227-37.

52. Dixon FJ, Weigle WO, Roberts JC. Comparison of antibody responses associated with the transfer of rabbit lymph node, peritoneal exudate and thymus cells. J Immunol 1957; 78: 56-60.

53. Billingham RE. Studies on the reaction of injected homologous lymphoid tissue cells against the host. Ann NY Acad Sci. 1958; 73: 782-89.

54. Billingham RE, Brent L. Quantitative studies on tissue transplantation immunity IV. Induction of tolerance in newborn mice and studies on the phenomenon of runt disease. Philos Trans R Soc London Ser B 1959; 242: 439-48.

55. Mori R, Nomoto K, Takeya K. Tumor formation by polyoma virus in neonatally thymectomized mice. Proc Jpn Acad 1964;40: 445-48.

56. Kirschten RL, Rabson AS, Peters LA. Oncogenic activity of adenovirus 12 in thymectomized BALB/c and C3H/HeN mice. Proc Soc Exp Biol Med 1964; 117: 198-202.

57. Law LW. Thymus: role in resistance to polyoma virus oncogenesis. Science 1965; 147: 164-67.

58. Law LW, Ting RC. Immunologic competence and induction of neoplasms by polyoma virus. Proc Soc Exp Biol Med 1965; 119: 823-31.

59. Law LW, Dunn TB, Trainen N, et al. Studies on thymic function. In:

Defendi V, Metcalf D, eds. The Thymus (Wistar Inst Symp Monogr No 2). Philadelphia: Wistar Institute Press, 1964: 105-27.

60. Azar HA, Snyder RW, Williams J. Dissociation between serum gamma globulin and precipitin antibody in rats thymectomized at birth. Fed Proc Fed Am Exp Biol 1963; 22: 600-07.

61. Azar HA, Williams J, Takasuki K. Development of plasma cells and immunoglobulins in neonatally thymectomized rats. In: Defendi V, Metcalf D, eds. The Thymus (Wistar Inst Symp Monogr No 2). Philadelphia: Wistar Institute Press, 1964: 75-116.

62. Humphrey JH. Studies on globulin and antibody production in mice thymectomized at birth. Proc R Soc Med 1964; 57: 151-54.

63. Humphrey JH, Parrott DMV, East J. Studies on globulin and antibody production in mice thymectomized at birth. Immunology 1964; 7: 419-27.

64. Fahey JL, Barth WF, Law LW. Normal immunolglobulins and antibody response in neonatally thymectomized mice. J Natl Cancer Inst 1965; 35: 663-70.

65. Arnason BG, de Vaux St. Cyr C, Grager P. Immunoglobulin abnormalities of the thymectomized rat. Nature 1963; 199: 1199-2002.

66. Miller JFAP. Immunological function of the thymus. Lancet 1961; 2: 748-51.

67. Miller JFAP. Effect of neonatal thymectomy on the immunological responsiveness of the mouse. Proc R Soc London Ser B 1961; 156: 415-21.

68. Schooley JC, Kelly BS. The thymus in lymphocyte production. Fed Proc Fed Am Soc Exp Biol 1961; 20: 71-75.

69. Miller JFAP. Immunity and the thymus. Lancet 1963; 1: 43-47.

70. Waksman BH, Arnason BG, Jankovic BD. Changes in the lymphoid organs of rats thymectomized at birth. Fed Proc Fed Am Soc Exp Biol 1962; 21: 274-84.

71. Sherman JD, Dameshek W. Wasting disease following thymectomy in the hamster. Nature 1963; 197: 469-72.

72. Archer OK, Pierce JC, Papermaster BW, et al. Reduced antibody responses in thymectomized rabbits. Nature 1962; 195: 191-93.

73. Claman HN, Talmage DW. Thymectomy: prolongation of immunological tolerance in the adult mouse. Science 1963; 142: 1193-96.

74. Law LW. Neoplasms in thymectomized mice following room infection with polyoma virus. Nature 1965; 205: 672-76.

75. Burnet M. Role of the thymus and related organs in immunity. Br Med J 1962; 3308: 807-11.

76. Rosen FS, Gitlin D, Janeway CA. Alymphocytosis, agammaglobulinemia, homografts and delayed hypersensitivity: Study of a case. Lancet 1962; 2: 380-83.

77. Miller JFAP, Ting RC, Law LW. Influence of thymectomy on tumor induction by polyoma virus in C57BL mice. Proc Soc Exp Biol Med 1964; 116: 123-31.

78. Sherman JD, Adner MM, Dameshek W. Effect of thymectomy on the golden hamster (Mesocricetus auratus). II. Studies of the immune response in thymectomized and splenectomized nonwasted animals. Blood 1964; 23: 375-84.

79. Salvin SB, Peterson RDA, Good RA. The role of the thymus in resistance to infection and endotoxin toxicity. J Lab Clin Med 1965; 65: 1004-10.

80. De Somer P, Denys P, Leyton R. Activity of noncellular thymus extract in normal and thymectomized mice. Life Sci 1963; 11: 810-15.

81. Burnett FM. Role of the thymus and related organs in immunity. Br Med J 1962; 2: 807-10.

82. Yohn DS, Funk CA Kalnins VI, Grace JT. Sex-related resistance in hamsters to adenovirus 12 oncogenesis. Influence of thymectomy at three weeks of age. J Natl Cancer Inst 1963; 35: 617-24.

83. Allison AC, Taylor RA. Observations on thymectomy and carcinogenesis. Cancer Res 1967; 27: 703-07.

84. Martinez C. Effect of early thymectomy on development of mammary tumors in mice. Nature 1964; 203: 1118-20.

85. Yunis EJH, Martinez EM, Smith J, et al. Spontaneous mammary adenocarcinoma in mice: influence of thymectomy and reconstitution with thymus grafts or spleen cells. Cancer Res 1969; 29: 174-77.

86. Moerttel GG. Multiple primary malignant neoplasms. Their incidence and significance. In: Moertel GG, ed. New York: Springer, 1972: 123-36.

87. Reinisch CL, Andrew SL, Schlossman SF. Suppressor cell regulation of immune response to tumors: abrogation by adult thymectomy. Proc Natl Acad Sci 1977; 74: 2989-92.

88. Olsson L, Ebbesen P, Hesse J. Influence of T-lymphocyte deprivation on the antileukemic effect of bacillus Calmette-Guérin in vivo. Cancer Immunol Immuother 1980; 8: 231-40.

89. Yoshimatsu H, Ishikura Y, Murakami M, et al. Clinical examination of thymic abnormalities and significance of thymectomy in patients with myasthenia gravis and other autoimmune diseases. J Uoeh 1979; 1: 487-505.

90. Takei F, Levy JG, Kilburn DG. Effect of adult thymectomy on adult tumor immunity in mice. Br J Cancer 1978; 37: 723-31.

91. Peer G, Paptestas AE, Tartter P, et al. Effects of thymectomy on mammary tumor growth. J Surg Res 1980; 28: 348-55.

92. Roubinian JR, Lane M, Slomich M, et al. Stimulation of immune mechanisms against mammary tumors in incomplete T-cell depletion. J Immunol 1976; 117: 1767-73.

93. Doll R, Kinlen L. Immunosurveillance and cancer: Epidemiological evidence. Br Med J 1970; 4: 420-22.

94. Vessey MP, Doll R. Thymectomy and cancer: follow-up study. Br J Cancer 1971; 26: 53-58.

95. Papatestas AE, Osserman KE, Kark AE. The relationship between thymus and oncogenesis. A study of the incidence of nonthymic malignancy in myasthenia gravis. Br J Cancer 1971; 25: 635-41.

96. Papatestas AE, Genkins G, Kornfeld P, et al. Transcervical thymectomy in myasthenia gravis. Surg Gynecol Obstet 1975; 140: 535-40.

97. Dean GO, Earle AM, Reilly WA. Failure of thymectomy in lymphatic leukemia. Arch Surg 1951; 63: 694-97.

98. Patey DH. A contribution to the study of Hodgkin's disease: late follow-up. Br J Surg 1980; 53: 387-89.

99. Surkovich SV, Dolestkii SI, Dul'tsin MS, et al. Thymectomy and X-ray of the thyroid gland in children with acute leukemia in the period of remission. Pediatria 1969; 48: 30-34.

100. Goldstein G, Mackay IR, eds. The Human Thymus. London: Heinemann, 1969: 304-25.

101. Itoh K, Maruchi N. Breast cancer in patients with Hashimoto's thyroiditis. Lancet 1975; 2: 1119-21.

CHAPTER 12

INDUCTION OF DONOR-SPECIFIC TRANSPLANTATION TOLERANCE WITH DIRECT INTRATHYMIC INJECTION OF SPLENOCYTE ALLOANTIGEN

Despite improvements in medical therapy, organ transplantation continues to be the only effective treatment for patients with isolated end-stage organ disease. However, Medawar[1] recognized early that an immunological reaction (rejection) directed against the transplantation antigen was the principle barrier to the ultimate success of this therapeutic approach. Rejection involves the recruitment and activation of CD4[+] helper T lymphocytes and the recognition and lysis of foreign cells by alloreactive CD8[+] cytotoxic T lymphocytes.[2] Pharmacologic advances in nonspecific immunosuppression and technical advances in solid organ transplantation have improved the survival results of kidney, liver, heart, lung and pancreas allografts over the last decade.[3,4] Although systemic immunosuppression for organ transplantation has improved considerably, its long-term use often results in drug toxicity and excessive immunosuppression continues as a major cause of morbidity and mortality for the transplant patient.[5,6] It has long been recognized that these complications could be avoided if it were possible to achieve a state of donor-specific unresponsiveness without subsequent immunosuppression as was described by Billingham et al[7] in the mouse neonatal tolerance model. The achievement of this state of tolerance appears to depend upon the presentation of antigen before the development of a competent T lymphocyte repertoire; thus allowing developing T cells to recognize the foreign antigen as self.

It is known that thymocytes originate from bone marrow multipotential hematopoietic stem cells and mature in the thymus into antigen reactive T lymphocytes before migrating to the peripheral lymphoid organs.[8,9] The T-cell receptors (TCR) expressed on T lymphocytes recognize foreign antigen physically associated with syngeneic cell surface products of the major histocompatibility complex (MHC).[10,11] By virtue of the heterodimeric αβ chains of the TCR, T cells recognize antigen in the context of self MHC encoded class I or class II molecules. CD4 and CD8 molecules, expressed

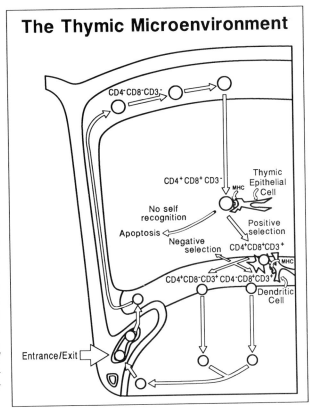

Fig. 1. Schematic view of the thymic microenvironment, demonstrating proposed regions of positive and negative selection events involved in thymocyte maturation and repertoire selection. [Modified from Boyd RL, Hugo P. An integrated view of thymopoiesis. Immunology Today 1991; 12(2): 72-73.]

on the surface of T lymphocytes bind to nonpolymorphic portions of the MHC class II and class I molecules respectively, and enhance the binding of the TCR to its ligand.[12,13] In the thymus (Fig. 1), precursors originating in the hematopoietic tissues undergo programmed proliferation, TCR gene rearrangement, differentiation, and repertoire selection. The development of TCR$^-$CD4$^-$CD8$^-$ T-cell precursors into TCR$^+$ cells expressing CD4 and/ or CD8 requires the presence of both MHC class II$^+$ epithelial cells and fetal mesenchyme.[14] Next, the differentiating thymocyte population is depleted of T cells possessing self-reactive TCR by apoptosis after interaction with intrathymic cells of the macrophage/dendritic cell lineage.[15-17] In contrast, immature T lymphocytes expressing T-cell receptors restricted to the recognition of foreign antigen in association with self-MHC class I and class II gene products are allowed to differentiate from CD4$^+$CD8$^+$ thymocytes into either CD4$^+$8$^-$ or CD4$^-$8$^+$ mature T lymphocytes.[18-20]

TOLERANCE SECONDARY TO INTRATHYMIC INJECTION OF CELLULAR ALLOANTIGEN

The concept of inducing tolerance with the intrathymic injection of allogeneic donor cells was initially reported in 1965 when Vojtiskova and Lengerova[21] demonstrated prolonged donor-specific H-3-disparate skin allograft survival. In this report, donor-specific tolerance was achieved when donor spleen cells were inoculated into an excised isogenic thymus which was then grafted under the skin in the thymic region of thymectomized recipients which had been sublethally irradiated (400 rads). The induction of tolerance was evaluated 13 weeks later by increased skin graft survival. Subsequently, Waksmann and colleagues[22-24] induced immune unresponsiveness to bovine γ-globulin by injecting this protein antigen directly into the shielded thymus of adult rats following sublethal total-body irradiation (800 rads). The thymus was essential to the development of tolerance in these experiments, since antigen injection at other sites (intraperitoneal and intrasplenic) did not result in tolerance induction. Additionally, Shimonkevitz and Bevan[25] have demonstrated that the transfer of semi-allogenic CD4/CD8 double-negative thymocyte stem cells into the thymus of irradiated host mice resulted in a transient state of chimerism in the host thymus, spleen and lymph nodes.

In the subsequent studies of Posselt et al,[26] Lewis (RT1^l) islets were transplanted into the thymus of diabetic Wistar-Furth (RT1^u) rats and simultaneously a single dose of rabbit anti-rat lymphocyte serum (ALS) was given peripherally. This protocol resulted in long-term (>100 days) survival of the transplanted islets and donor-specific tolerance to subsequent extrathymic islets allografts. Lymph node cells of the unresponsive recipients of intrathymic Lewis islets had a reduced (40-60%) precursor frequency of cytotoxic T lymphocytes (pCTL) to Lewis alloantigen while the pCTL for third-party alloantigen was not altered. These data suggested that deletion or functional inactivation of class I-restricted T lymphocytes to Lewis alloantigens had occurred.

We have recently extended these findings with intrathymic islet alloantigens by achieving indefinite, donor-specific, heterotopic cardiac allograft survival following pretransplant intrathymic injection of unfractionated splenocytes and a simultaneous single intraperitoneal injection of rabbit anti-rat lymphocyte serum.[27] By contrast, donor alloantigen injected at other sites did not prolong allograft survival.[27] We have also demonstrated that this induction of intrathymic tolerance is due to the intrathymic injection of MHC class II expressing spleen cells (B cells, macrophages, and dendritic cells)[28] while resting T lymphocytes and red blood cells (expressing only MHC class I) were not capable of tolerance induction. Additionally, we have shown that the intrathymic inoculum of donor allogeneic cells needs to consist of live cells, since freeze fractured and gamma irradiated (2000 rads) cells were not capable of inducing intrathymic tolerance (J.A.G. unpublished observation).[29]

EFFECT OF INTRATHYMIC DONOR SPLENOCYTE INJECTION ON CARDIAC ALLOGRAFT SURVIVAL

Donor-specific tolerance could be achieved (Table 1) for Lewis (RT1^l) heterotopic cardiac allografts[30] performed 21 days after the direct intrathymic injection of 25 x 10^6 unfractionated Lewis splenocytes and a simultaneous intraperitoneal injection of 1 ml ALS. The mean survival time of Lewis cardiac allografts in Buffalo (RT1^b) recipients receiving ALS alone or the intrathymic injection of Lewis splenocytes alone without ALS was 7.1 days, not significantly different from Buffalo recipients receiving no pretransplant treatment (mean survival time = 7.2 days) or a syngeneic intrathymic injection of Buffalo splenocytes followed by ALS (mean survival time = 6.8 days). However, intrathymic injection of fully allogeneic Lewis splenocytes plus intraperitoneal ALS resulted in indefinite Lewis cardiac allograft sur-

Table 1. Survival of Lewis or ACI heterotopic heart allografts in Buffalo rats

Group	Treatment	No. of Rats	Days of Survival	MST	p Value vs Controls
1	No treatment*	5	6,7,7,8,8	7.2	-
2	ALS or IT only*	8	6,6,7,7,7,7,8,9	7.1	NS
3	Buffalo IT + ALS*	6	6,6,7,7,7,8	6.8	NS
4	ACI IT + ALS (ACI Tx)	6	7,9,10,>100(x3)	>54.3	p<0.05
6	Lewis IT + ALS*	19	6,14,>100(x8),		
	>200(x8),>300	>176.8	p<0.001		
	2nd Heart (LEW)	4	>100 (x3),>200	>100.0	p<0.01
	2nd Heart (ACI)	3	7,7,7	7.0	NS

(*Groups receiving Lewis cardiac transplant)

vival (mean survival time >176.8 days, p<0.01 vs untreated controls) in 88% of Buffalo recipients. Donor-specific prolongation of cardiac allografts after intrathymic injection of cellular donor alloantigen and ALS is not limited to the Lewis/Buffalo strain combination, since ACI to Buffalo cardiac allograft survival was also markedly prolonged (mean survival time >54.3 days) after intrathymic injection of ACI splenocytes and a single intraperitoneal injection of ALS.[27]

Buffalo rats with long-term surviving Lewis cardiac allografts (>100 days) after Lewis intrathymic injection and a single dose of ALS rejected a heterotopic third-party ACI (RT1[a]) cardiac allograft in normal fashion (mean survival time = 7.0 days) (Table 1), whereas a second Lewis cardiac allograft was indefinitely accepted (mean survival time > 100.0 days), providing evidence that the induced tolerance was specific for the strain of donor cells given intrathymically.[31]

HISTOPATHOLOGIC ANALYSIS OF CARDIAC ALLOGRAFTS

Lewis cardiac allografts removed from Buffalo recipients receiving either no treatment, intrathymic injection of Lewis splenocytes alone, or ALS alone, at the time of cessation of contraction all demonstrated a typical dense mononuclear cell infiltration (Fig. 2a) and associated myofibril necrosis (Fig. 2b) consistent with an unmodified rejection response. In contrast, the beating Lewis cardiac allografts removed approximately 200 days after transplantation into a Buffalo recipient who previously had undergone intrathymic injection of Lewis alloantigen with ALS demonstrated healthy cardiac myocytes without mononuclear cell infiltration or evidence of tissue damage[27] (Fig. 2c).

LACK OF EFFECT OF INTRAVENOUS, INTRASPLENIC AND SUBCUTANEOUS SPLENOCYTE INJECTION ON CARDIAC ALLOGRAFT SURVIVAL

To determine whether the cellular alloantigen had to be placed within the thymus to induce this tolerance Buffalo recipients received pretransplant Lewis splenocytes via the intravenous, intrasplenic, and subcutaneous route

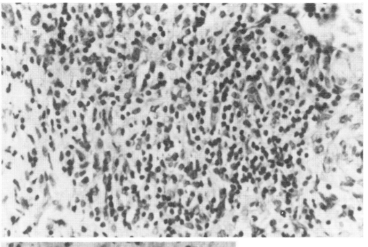

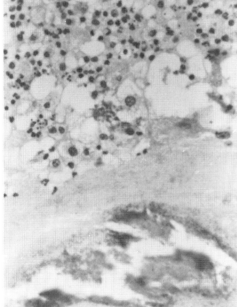

Fig. 2. Photomicrographs of Lewis cardiac allograft recovered from Buffalo recipients. (a, top) Section of a Lewis heart removed from an unmodified Buffalo recipient seven days after transplantation demonstrating a dense mononuclear cell infiltration (H&E 40x), and (b, left) associated myofibril necrosis (H&E 40x). (c, bottom) Section of a Lewis heart removed approximately 200 days after transplantation into a Buffalo recipient who previously had undergone an intrathymic injection of Lewis alloantigen and one dose of ALS, demonstrating healthy cardiac myocytes without mononuclear cell infiltration or evidence of tissue damage (H&E 40x).

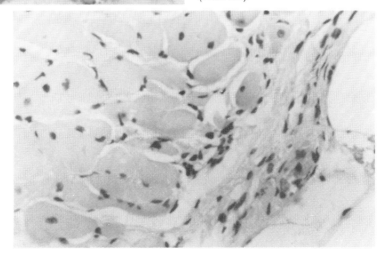

along with the single intraperitoneal injection of ALS 21 days before heterotopic Lewis cardiac allograft transplantation (Table 2). The mean survival time of Lewis cardiac allografts in Buffalo recipients who received Lewis alloantigen via the intravenous route plus ALS was 7.0 days, which is not significantly different from untreated control Buffalo recipients (MST = 7.2 days). All recipients receiving Lewis spleen cell alloantigen intrasplenically or subcutaneously rejected the heterotopic Lewis cardiac allograft by seven to nine days, which is also not significantly different from controls. These data suggest that the ability to produce a state of donor specific unresponsiveness needs the cellular alloantigen to be placed within the thymus where maturing T lymphocyte populations can be educated before replacing the peripheral T lymphocyte repertoire previously depleted by the administration of ALS.[27]

EFFECTS OF INTRATHYMIC ALLOANTIGEN ON DONOR CTL PRECURSOR FREQUENCY

The effect of intrathymic injection of Lewis splenocyte alloantigen on Buffalo anti-Lewis cytotoxic T lymphocyte (pCTL) precursor frequency was determined when spleen cells from Buffalo recipients with a long-term tolerated Lewis cardiac allograft, with an acutely rejecting cardiac allograft, or from naive Buffalo rats were serially compared by limiting dilution assay (LDA) for CTL precursor frequency. At all time points tested after transplantation, anti-Lewis pCTL was markedly decreased or absent in all Buffalo recipients who had a surviving Lewis cardiac allograft after intrathymic injection of Lewis alloantigen and a single injection of ALS (Table 3) while

Table 2. Survival of Lewis heart allografts in Buffalo rats

Group	Treatment	No. of Rats	Days of Survival	MST
7	IV inj. + ALS*	3	6,7,8	7.0
8	Intrasplenic inj. + ALS*	5	7,7,7,8,8	7.4
9	Subcutaneous inj. + ALS*	5	7,7,8,8,9	7.8

(*All groups received Lewis cardiac transplant)

Table 3. The effect of intrathymic Lewis alloantigen on recipient Buffalo pTH and pCTL

Days after Operation	pT Helper Cells*	Allospecific pCTL*
0 (Naive control)	1/22,900	1/99,830
7 (without Lew inj.)	1/18,600	1/47,998
7 (with Syn Buf inj.)†	1/12,680	1/7,780
3 (with Lew inj.)	1/90,339	<1/1,000,000
7 (with Lew inj.)	1/99,358	1/748,072
14 (with Lew inj.)	1/32,081	<1/1,000,000
40 (with Lew inj.)	1/74,572	<1/1,000,000
70 (with Lew inj.)	1/70,702	1/328,103
105 (with Lew inj.)	1/77,209	1/349,110

* pTH and pCTL obtained 7 days after Lewis cardiac transplant at the peak of rejection, 21 days after a syngeneic intrathymic Buffalo spleen cell injection.

Table 4. Proliferation to donor alloantigen after intrathymic transfer of Lewis splenocytes

Stimulators	[³H]Thymidine incorporation by responder cells from:					
	Lewis Alloantigen*			Naive Buffalo†		
	CPM	±	SD	CPM	±	SD
Medium only	937	±	117	789	±	104
Con A.	247,317	±	21,016	251,632	±	26,000
Lewis	97,141	±	7,431	95,647	±	8,623
ACI	169,314	±	12,609	172,017	±	14,011

* Spleen cells recovered from Long surviving Buffalo recipients 60 to 110 days after heterotopic Lewis cardiac allograft.
† Spleen cells recovered from a naive Buffalo rat.

third-party anti-ACI pCTL were not affected, e.g., 1/71,500 cells in Buffalo recipients with long-term surviving Lewis cardiac allograft vs. 1/75,100 cells in naive Buffalo animals. The CTL precursor frequency was increased in Buffalo animals who rejected the Lewis cardiac allograft (1/99,830 cells for naive Buffalo controls vs. 1/47,998 cells in Buffalo recipients acutely rejecting a Lewis cardiac allograft on posttransplant day 7).[27]

Nylon wool fractionated spleen cells from Buffalo recipients with long-term surviving Lewis cardiac allografts after intrathymic injection of Lewis alloantigen and from naive Buffalo rats were simultaneously evaluated for proliferation upon stimulation with Lewis or ACI alloantigen, or with Concanavalin A (10 µg/ml). Long-term surviving Buffalo recipient lymphocytes did not differ significantly from naive Buffalo spleen cells in their proliferative response to both donor (Lewis) or third-party (ACI) alloantigens or to Concanavalin A (Table 4). Additionally, the anti-Lewis T-helper lymphocyte (pTH) precursor frequency in these animals was moderately decreased (1/99,358 cells for Buffalo recipient tolerant of Lewis cardiac allografts vs. 1/22,900 cells for naive Buffalo controls) (Table 3). While pTH frequency to third-party ACI antigen did not change from control levels (1/24,200 vs. 1/22,900 cells, respectively).[27] These data suggest that a deletion or functional inactivation of cytotoxic but not proliferative T lymphocytes had occurred.

NECESSITY OF MHC CLASS II EXPRESSING CELLS

We next wanted to determine which donor MHC alloantigens must be injected intrathymically to induce this donor-specific tolerance to cardiac allografts. Lewis heterotopic cardiac allografts were performed 21 days after the intrathymic injection of fractionated Lewis donor cells and a simultaneous intraperitoneal injection of 1 ml of ALS. The mean survival time of Lewis cardiac allografts in Buffalo recipients receiving ALS treatment alone was 6.8 days (Table 5), which is not significantly different from Buffalo recipients receiving no pretransplant treatment (mean survival time = 7.5 days) or an intrathymic injection of unfractionated Lewis spleen cells without ALS (mean survival time = 6.2 days). Likewise, the pretransplant intrathymic injection of Lewis MHC class I only expressing red blood cells (purified by ficoll gradients) or resting T lymphocytes (purified by nylon wool)[28] did not significantly prolong Lewis cardiac allograft survival (mean survival time = 7.3 and 16.5 days, respectively). The prolonged Lewis cardiac allograft survival for one recipient in the T lymphocyte group is postulated to be secondary to contamination by class II expressing B lymphocyte, macrophage, or dendritic cells (Table 5). In contrast, intrathymic injection of enriched Lewis MHC class II expressing spleen cells (B lymphocytes, macrophages, and dendritic cells, purified by nylon wool and plastic adherence) plus ALS treatment resulted in significantly prolonged (mean survival time >125 days) Lewis cardiac allograft survival in all Buffalo recipients.[28] This data is similar to that obtained with intrathymic injection of unfractionated splenocytes[27] (Tables 1 and 5) and indicates that the ability to produce a state of donor-specific unresponsiveness requires that MHC class II expressing cells be placed within the thymus.

Donor-specificity was again documented when Buffalo recipients tolerant to Lewis cardiac allografts underwent a second ACI or Lewis heterotopic cardiac transplant. Buffalo rats with a long-surviving Lewis cardiac allograft rejected a third-party ACI cardiac allograft in normal fashion (mean survival time = 7.0 days), while a second Lewis cardiac allograft was accepted indefinitely (mean survival time > 100.0 days) (Table 6).[28]

Table 5. Influence of splenocyte cell fraction on survival of Lewis heterotopic heart allografts into Buffalo rats

Group	Pretransplant Treatment*	No. of Rats	Days of Survival	MST	p Value vs Control
1	No treatment	6	7,7,7,8,8,8	7.5	—
2	ALS only	6	6,6,7,7,7,8	6.8	NS
3	IT inj. only	6	5,6,6,6,7,7	6.2	NS
4	RBC IT + ALS	6	7,7,7,7,8,8	7.3	NS
5	T cell IT + ALS	6	7,7,8,8,9,>60	16.5	NS
6	(B cell, macrophage dendritic) adherent cells IT + ALS[x]	6	>100(x3), >150(x3)	>125.0	p<0.001 vs Group 1
	Unfrac. spleen cell + IT	25	6,7,14,>100(x6), >200(x16)	>153.1	p<0.001 vs Group 1

* Heterotopic Lewis cardiac grafts were placed 21 days after pretreatment
[x] Splenocytes adherent to plastic dishes were >90% B cells, macrophages and dendritic cells

Table 6. Second allograft survival in long-term Lewis heart bearing Buffalo rats

Allograft	Second Allograft Survival Time (days)
Heart (ACI)	7,7,7
Heart (Lewis)	>100, >100, >100

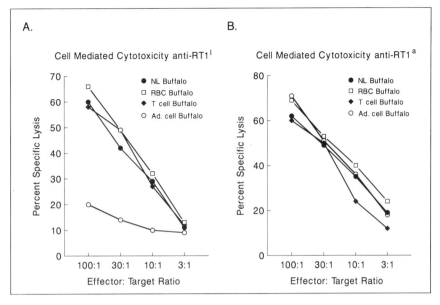

Fig. 3. Intrathymic injection of Lewis MHC class II expressing cells, with ALS, specifically inhibits the in vitro Buffalo anti-Lewis cytotoxic response. (a) Primary Buffalo anti-Lewis specific CTL were assayed against AS-F4 (RT1^l) targets following the intrathymic injection of MHC class II expressing B cells, macrophages, and dendritic cells (○), MHC class I expressing red blood cells (□), MHC class I expressing resting T lymphocytes (●). Controls also include naive, nonthymic injected Lewis-specific Buffalo effector cells (◆). (b) ACI (RT1^a) specific CTL were analyzed following the intrathymic injection of the same cell population as in Fig. 3a. Additionally, ACI specific effectors were generated from naive Buffalo responders. All effectors were tested against Concanavalin A blasted ACI lymphocytes. [From Goss JA, et al. MHC class II presenting cells are necessary for the induction of intrathymic tolerance. Ann Surg 1993; 217: 497.]

These in vivo studies were expanded when lymph node cells harvested from either Buffalo recipients with a long-term tolerated Lewis cardiac allograft after MHC class II intrathymic injection, from an acutely rejecting Lewis cardiac following the intrathymic injection of MHC class I alloantigens, or from nontransplanted naive Buffalo rats were analyzed for Lewis- and ACI-specific cell mediated cytotoxicity. The intrathymic injection of Lewis MHC class II expressing cells, with ALS, resulted in a marked decrease in the anti-RT1^l (Lewis) cytolytic response in contrast to the strong cytolytic activity against the RT1^l targets by naive control, or Lewis MHC class I intrathymically injected Buffalo recipients (Fig. 3a). The intrathymic injection of Lewis MHC class II expressing cells did not alter the anti-RT1^a (ACI) third-party response when compared to naive controls or MHC class I injected recipients (Fig. 3b). These data demonstrated that the intrathymic injection of Lewis MHC class II expressing cells specifically induce tolerance only to the donor strain injected intrathymically, and does not globally immunosuppress the host.

The lymph node cells harvested from Buffalo recipients following the intrathymic injection of Lewis MHC class II or class I expressing cells, or no pretransplant treatment were also analyzed for their production of interleukin (IL)-2 during stimulation with irradiated (2000 rads) Lewis or ACI

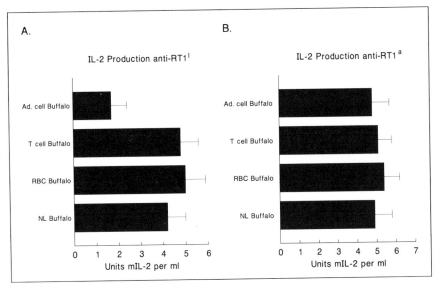

Fig. 4. Inhibition of Lewis-specific IL-2 production following the intrathymic injection of MHC class II expressing Lewis allogeneic cells. (a) Supernatants from Buffalo anti-Lewis mixed lymphocyte cultures were harvested after 48 hours and analyzed for IL-2. Buffalo recipients underwent the intrathymic injection of Lewis MHC class II adherent cells, Lewis red blood cells, resting Lewis T lymphocytes, or no pretreatment. Only recipients receiving Lewis adherent cells had decreased IL-2 production. (b) Buffalo anti-ACI 48 hour mixed lymphocyte culture supernatant was analyzed for IL-2 production from Buffalo recipients of intrathymic Lewis MHC class II adherent cells, red blood cells, resting T lymphocytes, or no pretransplant treatment. [From Goss JA, et al. MHC class II presenting cells are necessary for the induction of intrathymic tolerance. Ann Surg 1993; 217: 497.]

lymph node cells. Buffalo lymph node cells harvested from the recipients undergoing the pretransplant intrathymic injection of Lewis MHC class II expressing allogeneic cells with ALS produced 50% less IL-2 upon stimulation with Lewis lymph node cells when compared to naive and Lewis MHC class I injected Buffalo recipients (Fig. 4a). However, the intrathymic injection of Lewis MHC class II expressing cells did not alter the recipients IL-2 production to a third-party ACI lymph node stimulation (Fig. 4b).

TIMING OF INDUCTION OF INTRATHYMIC TOLERANCE

Subsequent experiments attempted to outline the kinetics of tolerance induction following the direct intrathymic inoculation of MHC class II expressing spleen cells.[32] In these experiments the Buffalo recipient underwent an intrathymic injection with 25×10^6 spleen cells and a simultaneous intraperitoneal injection of ALS on day 0. This was followed by total thymectomy one, three and seven days later and finally the performance of a heterotopic Lewis cardiac transplant on postintrathymic injection day 21. As is outlined in Table 7, Buffalo recipients receiving no pretransplant treatment rejected Lewis cardiac allografts within eight days (mean survival time = 7.4 days). As previously shown the intrathymic injection of Lewis splenocytes plus a single dose of ALS resulted in a dramatically prolonged Lewis cardiac allograft survival (mean survival time >77.0 days). Thymectomy one and three days after Lewis spleen cell injection did not change the normal rejection time of Lewis cardiac allografts (mean survival times = 6.8 and 8.0 days, respectively) indicating that removal of the thymus at these time points prevented the development of tolerance. In contrast, thymectomy seven days after intrathymic Lewis spleen cell injection resulted in indefinite prolongation of Lewis cardiac allograft survival in 75% of the recipients evaluated (mean survival time >77.0 days).[32] These data demonstrate that cellular donor alloantigen must be present in the thymus for approximately seven days to induce this type of donor-specific unresponsiveness which allows the indefinite survival of a fully allogeneic vascularized graft. Additional control experiments were performed to rule out the possibility that thymectomy alone or in combination with alloantigen injected at other sites with ALS may prolong allograft survival. As shown in Table-8, thymectomy alone, 14 days before cardiac transplantation, after either no treatment, ALS intraperitoneally only, or after the intravenous injection of 25×10^6 Lewis spleen cells with ALS intraperitoneally did not prolong Lewis cardiac allograft survival. These data verify that the prolonged cardiac allograft survival was the result of intrathymic injection of cellular alloantigen and not the nonspecific immunosuppressive effects of thymectomy and ALS.[32]

Tissue-Specific Tolerance

To determine whether the intrathymic injection of splenocyte alloantigen plus a single dose of ALS could induce tolerance to other organ allografts, 25×10^6 donor Lewis splenocytes were injected intrathymically and a intraperitoneal injection of ALS was given 21 days before the Buffalo recipient received a Lewis renal or full thickness abdominal skin allograft.[33]

Table 7. Effect of timing of thymectomy after intrathymic injection of Lewis splenocytes with ALS treatment on Lewis cardiac allograft survival in Buffalo rats

Group	Pretreatment	Thymectomy	Days of Survival	MST	p value vs Group 1
1	None	ND	7,7,7,8,8	7.4	—
2	IT + ALS	ND	6,7,14,>100(x22)	>89.1	p<0.001
3	IT + ALS	day 1	6,7,7,7,7	6.8	NS
4	IT + ALS	day 3	7,7,8,8,8,10	8.0	NS
5	IT + ALS	day 7	6,10,>100(x6)	>77.0	p<0.001

Table 8. Effect of thymectomy alone or combined with other treatments on Lewis cardiac allograft survival in Buffalo rats

Group	Pretreatment	Thymectomy	Days of Survival	MST	p value vs Group 1
1	None	ND	7,7,7,8,8	7.4	—
6	None	day 7	7,7,7,7	7.0	NS
7	ALS	day 7	7,7,7,8,9	7.6	NS
8	IV + ALS	day 7	7,8,8,10	8.3	NS

The mean survival time of Lewis renal allografts in Buffalo recipients receiving ALS treatment alone was 7.6 days, which is not significantly different from recipients receiving no pretransplant treatment (mean survival time = 7.8 days) (Table 9). Intrathymic injection of unfractionated allogeneic Lewis splenocytes plus a single dose of ALS resulted in prolonged renal allograft survival (mean survival time = 14.8 days) but did not result in indefinite renal allograft survival as was found in the cardiac allograft experiments.[27,28,31,32,33] Additionally, the intrathymic injection of unfractionated allogeneic Lewis spleen cells and a single dose of ALS did not significantly prolong skin allograft survival (Table 9).

Additional experiments were performed to determine the cause for this inability to produce tolerance for these two organs. As shown in Table 10,

Table 9. Lewis allograft survival in Buffalo rats injected with 25x10⁶ splenocytes intrathymically and/or ALS intraperitoneally 21 days before transplantation

Group	TREATMENT IT	ALS	Allograft from LEW	Survival Time (days)	MST	p value
1	-	-	Heart	7,7,7,8,8	7.4	—
2	-	+	Heart	6,7,7,7,8,9	7.3	NS
3	+ (LEW)	-	Heart	5,6,6,6,7	6.0	NS
4	+ (LEW)	+	Heart	6,7,14, >100(x6), >200(x16)	>153.1	p<0.001
5	-	-	Kidney	7,7,7,8,9,9	7.8	—
6	-	+	Kidney	7,7,8,8,8	7.6	NS
7	+ (LEW)	+	Kidney	10,14,15,17,18	14.8	p<0.05
8	-	-	Skin	8,9,9,10,10	9.2	—
9	-	+	Skin	9,9,9,10,10	9.4	NS
10	+ (LEW)	+	Skin	10,11,12,12,13	11.6	NS

Table 10. Second allograft survival in long-term Lewis heart bearing Buffalo rats and the course of first Lewis cardiac allografts

Group	Allograft	2nd Allograft Survival Time (days)	1st Lewis Cardiac Allograft Survival Time (days)
4a	Heart (LEW)	>100,>100,>100	>100,>100,>100
4b	Heart (ACI)	7,7,7	>100,>100,>100
4c-1	Kidney (LEW)	17,18,18	>17†,>18†,>18†
4c-2	Kidney (LEW)#	10*,10*,10*	>100§,>100§,>100§
4d	Skin (LEW)	9,10,11	>100§,>100§,>100§

#No contralateral nephrectomy
*Nephrectomy of transplanted kidney was performed 10 days after renal transplantation. Rejection was confirmed by histologic examination
**First Lewis cardiac allograft survival time after second allograft transplantation
†Functioning at death
§First Lewis cardiac allografts were retransplanted into naive Buffalo rats

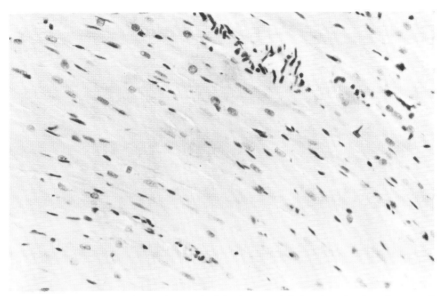

Fig. 5. Long-term accepted Lewis heart which had survived during the rejection of a second Lewis renal allograft, removed 120 days after kidney transplantation. There are healthy cardiac myocytes and neither evidence of rejection nor tissue damage (H&E, original magnification 160x).

Table 11. Survival of retransplanted long-surviving Lewis cardiac allografts into naive Buffalo recipients

Group	Graft	Survival Time (days)	MST
1	Naive LEW heart	7,7,7,8,8	7.4
11	Long-surviving LEW cardiac allograft (in Buffalo)	7,7,7	7.0

Buffalo recipients with long-term surviving Lewis cardiac allografts after the intrathymic injection of Lewis spleen cells and ALS underwent a second Lewis renal[34,35] or skin[36] allograft. Both the Lewis skin and renal allografts were rejected in a prolonged fashion (Table 10), but it is noteworthy that the rejection of these organs did not cause any clinical or histological evidence of rejection in the cardiac allograft (Fig. 5). To rule out the possibility that cardiac allograft acceptance, despite renal and skin allograft rejection, was secondary to the cardiac allograft having lost its immunogenicity, three long-term surviving Lewis cardiac allografts removed from the recipient more than 100 days after transplantation and retransplanted into naive Buffalo recipients were all rejected in a normal fashion (Table 11).[33] Therefore it would appear that the skin[37,38] and kidney[39-42] possess tissue-specific antigens to which these rejection episodes were directed which are not present on the heart or the spleen cell population that is inoculated into the thymus for the induction of tolerance.

Summary

Our findings suggest that the presence of directly intrathymically injected allogeneic splenocyte MHC class II antigens into the adult thymic microenvironment during thymocyte maturation, following a brief period of immunosuppression, has a markedly different effect, i.e., graft acceptance and reduction of cytolytic T lymphocytes, than when donor alloantigen is placed in a site other than the thymus. The achievement of indefinite donor-specific allograft survival in mature adult rats and the reduction of donor-specific pCTL after intrathymic injection of the donor splenocyte alloantigens demonstrates that the adult thymic environment can be manipulated to result in the development of tissue-specific, donor-specific tolerance across a full MHC barrier. Previously it was shown that transplantation of an allogeneic thymus or intrathymic inoculation of semi-allogeneic thymic stem cells into lethally irradiated mice reconstituted with syngeneic bone marrow could induce tolerance in the recipient to the donor alloantigen.[43,44] In addition, it has been shown that mice transgeneic for T-cell receptors that react to specific peptide antigens produce tolerance to that antigen by deleting thymocytes reactive to the specific peptide antigens within the thymic medulla at the CD4[+]CD8[+] developmental stage.[45,46] These findings are consistent with the recent report that thymic antigen presenting cells are capable of presenting exogenous antigen in association with MHC class I but not class II molecules, and have implications for the repertoire of peptides that are displayed to developing T cells.[47]

In conclusion, we have demonstrated that the direct intrathymic injection of MHC class II expressing splenocyte alloantigen plus a single simultaneous injection of ALS induces indefinite tolerance to donor-specific cardiac allografts if the thymus is left in place for at least seven days—but not to renal or skin allografts. Additionally, a second renal or skin allograft of the same strain is rejected even when subsequently placed into a recipient with a long-term surviving cardiac allograft, suggesting that the rejection of these organs occurs because of the presence of non-MHC tissue-specific antigens.

References

1. Medawar PB. The behavior and fate of skin allografts and skin homografts in rabbits. J Anat 1944; 78: 176-87.
2. Krensky A, Weiss A, Crabtree G, et al. T lymphocyte-antigen interactions in transplant rejection. N Engl J Med 1990; 322: 510-16.
3. Bach FH, Sachs DH. Transplantation immunology. N Engl J Med 1987; 318: 645-48.
4. Foker JE, Simmons RL, Najarian JS. Recent advances in transplantation. In: Najarian JS, Simmons RL, eds. Allograft Rejection. Philadelphia: Lea Febringer, 1972: 63-145.
5. Kahan BD. Cyclosporine. N Engl J Med 1989; 321: 1725-33.
6. Walker RG, d'Apice AJF. Azathioprine and Steroids. In: Morris PJ, ed. Kidney Transplantation: Principles and Practices. Philadelphia: WB Saunders, 1988: 319-41.
7. Billingham RL, Brent L, Medawar PB. Actively acquired tolerance to foreign cells. Nature 1953; 172: 603-06.
8. Miller JFAP, Marshall A, White R. The immunological significance of the thymus. Adv Immunol 1962; 2: 111-48.

9. Adkins G, Mueller C, Okada C, et al. Early events in T-cell maturation. Ann Rev Immunol 1987; 5: 325-56.

10. Babbit B, Allen P, Matsueda G, et al. Binding of immunogenic peptides to Ia histocompatibility molecules. Nature 1985; 317: 359-63.

11. Bjorkman P, Saper M, Samraoui B, et al. The foreign antigen binding site and T-cell recognition regions of class I histocompatibility antigens. Nature 1987; 324: 512-16.

12. Gabert J, Langlet C, Zamoyska R, et al. Reconstitution of MHC class I specificity by transfer of the T-cell receptor and Lyt-2 genes. Cell 1987; 50: 545-54.

13. Gay D, Maddon P, Sekaly R, et al. Functional interaction between human T-cell protein CD4 and the major histocompatibility complex HLA-DR antigen. Nature 1987; 328: 626-29.

14. Anderson G, Jenkinson EJ, Moore NC, et al. MHC class II-positive epithelium and mesenchyme cells are both required for T-cell development in the thymus. Nature 1993; 362: 70-72.

15. Longo D, Schwartz R. T-cell specificity for H-2 and Ir gene phenotype correlates with the phenotype of thymic antigen-presenting cells. Nature 1980; 287: 44-47.

16. Ready A, Jenkinson E, Kingston R, et al. Successful transplantation across major histocompatibility barrier of deoxyguanosine-treated embryonic thymus expressing class II antigens. Nature 1984; 310: 231-33.

17. Longo D, Davis M. Early appearance of donor-type antigen-presenting cells in the thymuses of 1200 R radiation-induced bone marrow chimeras correlates with self-recognition of donor I region gene products. J Immunol 1983; 130: 2525-31.

18. Teh HS, Kisielow P, Scott B. Thymic major histocompatibility complex antigens and the alpha beta T-cell receptor determine the CD4/CD8 phenotype of T cells. Nature 1988; 335: 229-32.

19. Bevan MJ. In a radiation chimera host, H-2 antigens determine the immune responsiveness of donor cytotoxic cells. Nature 1977; 269: 417-20.

20. Zinkernagel R, Callahan G, Althage A, et al. The lymphoreticular system in triggering virus plus self-specific cytotoxic T cells: Evidence for T-cell help? J Exp Med 1978; 147: 882-91.

21. Vojtiskova M, Lengerova A. On the possibility that thymus-mediated alloantigenic stimulation results in tolerance response. Experientia 1965; 21: 661-63.

22. Staples PJ, Gery I, Waksman BH. Role of the thymus in tolerance: III. Tolerance to bovine gamma globulin after direct injections of antigen into the shielded thymus of irradiated rats. J Exp Med 1966; 124: 127-39.

23. Gery I, Waksman BH. Role of the thymus in tolerance: V. Suppressive effect of treatment with nonaggregated and aggregated bovine gamma globulin in specific immune responses in normal adult rats. J Immunol 1967; 98: 446-50.

24. Horiuchi A, Waksman BH. Role of the thymus in tolerance: VI. Tolerance to bovine gamma globulin in rats given low doses of irradiation and injection of nonaggregated or aggregated antigen into the shielded thymus. J Immunol 1968; 100: 974-78.

25. Shimonkevitz R, Bevan M. Split tolerance induced by the intrathymic adoptive transfer of thymocyte stem cells. J Exp Med 1988; 168: 143-56.

26. Posselt AM, Barker CF, Tomaszewski JA, et al. Induction of donor-specific

unresponsiveness by intrathymic islet transplantation. Science 1990; 249: 1293-95.

27. Goss JA, Nakafusa Y, Flye MW. Intrathymic injection of donor alloantigens induces specific tolerance to cardiac allografts. Transplantation 1993; 56: 166-73.

28. Goss JA, Nakafusa Y, Flye MW. MHC class II presenting cells are necessary for the induction of intrathymic tolerance. Ann Surg 1993; 217: 492-99.

29. Odorico JS, Barker CF, Posselt AM, et al. Induction of donor-specific tolerance to rat cardiac allografts by intrathymic inoculation of bone marrow. Surgery 1992; 112: 370-77.

30. Ono K, Lindsey ES. Improved technique of heart transplantation in rats. J Thorac Cardiovasc Surg 1969; 57: 225-31.

31. Goss JA, Nakafusa Y, Flye MW. Donor-specific cardiac allograft tolerance without immunosuppression after intrathymic injection of donor alloantigen. Transplant Proc 1992; 24: 2879-80.

32. Nakafusa Y, Goss JA, Flye MW. Prevention by thymectomy of tolerance induced by intrathymic injection of donor splenocytes. Surgery 1993; 114: 183-89.

33. Nakafusa Y, Goss JA, Flye MW. Intrathymic injection of splenocyte alloantigen induces donor specific tolerance to cardiac but not skin or renal allografts. Transplantation 1993; 55: 877-82.

34. Kamada N. A description of cuff techniques for renal transplantation in the rat. Transplantation 1985; 39: 93-98.

35. Savas CP, Nolan MS, Lindsey NJ, et al. Renal transplantation in the rat: A new simple, non suture technique. Urol Res 1985; 13: 91-96.

36. Billingham RE. Free skin grafting in mammals. In: Billingham RE, Silver WK, eds. Transplantation of Tissues and Cells. Philadelphia: Wistar Institute, 1961: 1-25.

37. Steinmuller D. Tissue-specific and tissue-restricted histocompatibility antigens. Immunology Today 1984; 5: 234-47.

38. Burlingham WJ, Steinmuller D. Cell-mediated cytotoxicity to nonmajor histocompatibility complex alloantigens on mouse epidermal cells. Transplantation 1983; 35: 130-35.

39. Carpenter CC, d'Apice AJF, Abbas AK. The role of antibodies in the rejection and enhancement of organ allografts. Adv Immunol 1976; 22: 1-24.

40. Vegt PA, Buurman WA, van der Linden CJ, et al. Cell-mediated cytotoxicity toward canine kidney epithelial cells. Transplantation 1982; 33: 465-70.

41. Mohanakumar T, Phibbs M, Haar J, et al. Alloantibodies eluted from rejected human renal allografts. Reactivity to primary kidney cells in culture. Transplantation Proc 1980; 12: 65-68.

42. Masmimo S, Sakai A, Ochiai T, et al. The mixed kidney cell-lymphocyte reaction in rats. Tissue Antigens 1976; 7: 291-98.

43. Lo D, Sprent J. Identity of cells that imprint H-2 restricted T-cell specificity in the thymus. Nature 1986; 319: 672-75.

44. Saluan J, Bandeira A, Khazaal I, et al. Thymic epithelium tolerizes for histocompatibility antigens. Science 1990; 247: 1471-74.

45. Murphy KM, Meimberger AB, Loh DY. Induction by antigen of intrathymic apoptosis of CD4+CD8+ TCR thymocytes in vivo. Science 1990; 250: 1720-23.

46. Swat W, Ignatowicz L, von Boehmer H, et al. Clonal deletion of immature CD4+ CD8+ thymocytes in suspension culture by extrathymic antigen presenting cells. Nature 1991; 350: 150.

47. Grant EP, Rock KL. MHC class I restricted presentation of exogenous antigen by thymic antigen-presenting cells in vitro and in vivo. J Immunol 1992; 148: 13-19.

INDEX